LEARNING TO EAT

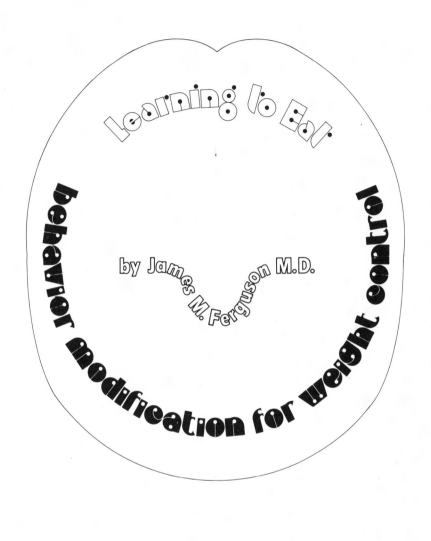

Learning to Eat:

behavior modification for weight control

by James M. Ferguson M.D.

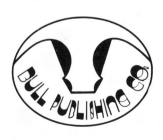

BULL PUBLISHING CO.

P.O. Box 208, Palo Alto, CA 94301

ISBN 0-915950-02-2

CONTENTS

INTRODUCTION

Lesson One
INTRODUCTION TO THE BEHAVIORAL CONTROL OF WEIGHT—
HABIT AWARENESS

Lesson Two
CUE ELIMINATION

Lesson Three
CHANGING THE ACT OF EATING

Lesson Four
BEHAVIOR CHAINS AND ALTERNATE ACTIVITIES

Lesson Five
BEHAVIORAL ANALYSIS, PROGRESS, AND PROBLEM SOLVING

MAINTENANCE WEEK—5

Lesson Six
PRE-PLANNING

Lesson Seven
CUE ELIMINATION, PART TWO AND ENERGY USE, PART ONE

Lesson Eight
ENERGY USE, PART TWO

Lesson Nine
SNACKS, CUES AND HOLIDAYS

Lesson Ten
ENVIRONMENTAL SUPPORT—FAMILY AND FRIENDS

BIBLIOGRAPHY

The individual techniques in this manual have been collected from many sources. In most cases, it is impossible to say who first thought of each individual therapeutic technique, and award credit accordingly. Food diaries, self monitoring, behavioral analysis, increasing activity, decreasing cue saliency, snack substitution, decreasing rate of eating, reinforcement for homework and attendance, feedback about progress, and family interventions are the stock in trade of modern nutritional counseling.

The work of the following investigators in the areas indicated was relied on as source material for this manual.

C.B. Ferster is one of the pioneers in obesity research who looked into the psychological determinants of eating behaviors and proposed the model from which ultimately this program has been derived.

R.L. Hagen has explored the role of bibliotherapy and aversive treatments in weight control programs.

H.A. Jordan has developed materials for use in behavioral weight reduction programs, along with investigating the determinants of hunger and satiety in the thin and obese populations.

L.S. Levitz has worked with weight control program development and self help programs for the obese.

M.J. Mahoney has extensively investigated the cognitive aspects of hunger, eating, and satiety, and has systematically explored the basic postulates underlying the behavioral treatments of obesity.

J.E. Mayer demonstrated much of the basic physiology of eating and the relationship between activity levels and obesity.

W.T. McReynolds has investigated the elements of behavior therapy programs for weight control and has developed stimulus control techniques to the ultimate (e.g., removing light bulbs from patients' refrigerators).

R.E. Nesbett extensively investigated the cognitive aspects of eating behaviors and the cues for hunger and satiety.

S.B. Penick demonstrated the efficacy of behavioral methods and the worth of groups for treating obesity.

L.D. Ross investigated cue saliency and developed some of the common sense "out of sight, out of mind" cue elimination techniques.

S. Schacter devised many brilliant experiments to illustrate the effects of the environment on the eating response in humans.

R.B. Stuart is the experimenter and organizer par excellence of the field of obesity and weight control.

A.J. Stunkard has been both an experimenter and key theoretician in weight control for the past twenty-five years.

J.P. Wollersheim was the first person to investigate the effect of a written program like Learning to Eat in group therapy situations.

Susan and Orland Wooley have carried out one of the most systematic series of investigations into the mechanisms of hunger, satiety, and eating behavior.

P. Watslowick, J. Haley, S. Minuchin, and G. Bach have been my models for family and couple interaction and intervention as described in the final chapter.

INTRODUCTION

This manual is for your use in a behavioral weight control program. It is written to accompany the presentation of your group leader (or therapist) during the weekly lessons. You are encouraged to take notes on the outlines in this manual, and to underline points which are significant to you or which have special meaning to your life situation.

The outline for each week will closely follow the verbal presentation of your group leader. If you do not understand any of the materials presented by your leader or in the outline, ask your leader for help. It is necessary for you to have a good understanding of the theory and homework presented at each lesson if you are going to change your eating behaviors.

This manual was initially written for the Stanford University Eating Disorders Clinic. It is based on theories developed in many different areas of psychology, and, if used as written, will be quite effective in helping you control your eating behaviors. Most people find the manual continues to be useful long after the behavior change program is over. If, three months, a year, or five years from now, you find your eating behaviors are getting out of control, take out your manual, fill out a Food Diary for a few weeks, and choose the appropriate techniques to correct whatever problems are leading to over-eating. They will be as valid five years from now as they are today.

Many of the exercises presented in the program may seem tedious or dull. We urge you to try them all and to give each one a good personal evaluation before you discard it. Success in changing eating patterns goes along with a willingness to try each new technique and fit it into your life.

There are few predictors of who will do well and who will do poorly in this group. Out of every ten people who enter the program, two will probably not do well. (Figure 1) Regular attendance and completion of all the homework are hallmarks of success in the program. This is because you can only be successful if you apply the techniques. Once you are successful, you will feel more like trying additional techniques.

If you are going to miss a meeting for any reason, tell your group leader in advance. He or she can help you with an alternate weighing time, and perhaps can see you individually to make up for the missed lesson.

During the course, be on the lookout for rationalizations in yourself and others which lead to a lessening of motivation. You can easily spot them, in statements like, "I only ate spinach for a week and gained four pounds, I must be different...," or, "I could never give up my morning newspaper while I am eating my eggs and bacon...," or, "These are great techniques, but they don't apply to me." If you establish the habit of saying, "yes, but...," it is virtually guaranteed that you will not be successful in this program.

Each lesson will be held in a group. It is important to understand that these are not psychotherapy groups. We have no intention of revealing personal secrets or confidential information. In the group we will treat an individual's weight and gain or loss as confidential. If you wish to share this information, it will be your decision. There will be no pigs or turtles to wear, no humiliation or testimonials, no songs or slogans, and only whatever minimal emphasis you want to place on competition.

FIGURE 1. WEEKLY WEIGHT LOSS FOR INDIVIDUAL MEMBERS OF A BEHAVIORAL WEIGHT CONTROL GROUP

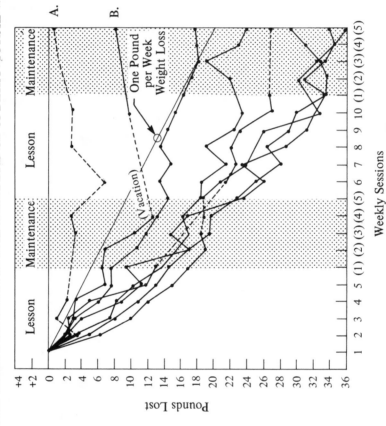

Each group member is represented by one line. Broken lines indicate missed meetings, and shaded areas represent Maintenance weeks. Patient A was a businessman who could not attend meetings regularly; Patient B went on vacation during the second half of the course. This graph is easier to prepare and read if you use a different color for each group member. This week-to-week graph will help you keep track of each individual's progress in relation to the rest of their group.

If the group desires, you can vote to abandon your weight confidentiality and compare your weights. This is a decision for the group and not the group leader and, in any event, you will not be forced to divulge information unless you want to. If you do share weight change information, keep in mind that competition can be destructive as well as constructive. If you feel it will not help you, it is probably best to simply compare yourself with the group average, without joining in the exchange of weight information.

This behavior therapy group is a learning situation like a school class. It is a course devoted to learning new eating behaviors. We meet in groups because this is the best way to learn. Within the group there is mutual support, public commitment, and a chance to share successes with other people.

Many people entering a weight control group are frightened because they have heard tales of wild encounter and psychotherapy groups. In this group, we are not interested in increasing sensitivity or discussing emotions. We will remain task oriented. The task is to learn new eating behaviors.

We recommend that everyone entering the program has had a recent physical examination by their physician. Although it is very rare (less than one percent of overweight patients) to have a physical cause for obesity, everyone should make sure before they begin a weight control program. Female members of the group should remember that a loss of weight is often accompanied by an increase in fertility and in some cases by a resumption of menses. If at the present time your weight is preventing you from being fertile, you may want to see your physician for birth control advice before you lose too much weight.

This program is not a diet and does not contain dietary instruction. If you want to restrict your caloric intake while you are changing your eating behaviors, many commercial diets are available. They will accelerate your rate of weight loss. The diets recommended are those of the American Heart Association, and those available from your physician or a consulting dietician. In no case should diets be lower than 1200 calories unless under supervision. Very low-caloric diets are usually accompanied by depression and a feeling of restriction and guilt about eating. One of the objects of this program is to escape from the feeling of guilt and punishment associated with food restriction. Food is to be enjoyed, and enjoyment can only come when you feel in control of your eating and confident that you can eat whatever you want in moderation.

You have been asked to pay for your treatment in advance. The reasons for this are not entirely financial. Pre-payment increases attendance and decreases the number of drop-outs. Because this is a learning program, each lesson missed is a week's instruction missed. You must learn the entire program to have your best chance of success.

We have also collected a refundable deposit from you. Your money will be returned to you for completing your homework. The quality of homework, spelling, neatness, etc. will not be considered. What we are interested in is simply the completed homework. A Homework Credit schedule is included in this manual, showing the schedule of repayment.

Our experience shows that those of you who are successful will be those who don't miss weekly meetings, the motivated people who complete all the homework and try all of the techniques. This is why the refund has been built into the program, rewarding you with money for completing your homework. Eventually, your home environment will take over the function of rewarding you for behavior change, in the form of compliments on your looks, greater mobility, sense of freedom—a good feeling about yourself.

Many of you have had unpleasant experiences revealing your weight to family and friends and in front of previous groups. We do not want to repeat these bad feelings or have you view us or the process of being weighed as punishment. In this program you will be weighed each week. The scale will be an impartial tool which gives us feedback about your success, and our success in helping you change your behaviors. We're in this together.

If your weight loss is slow, remember that everyone loses at his or her own rate: Individuals with childhood onset of obesity may lose more slowly than those who became overweight as adults. Men often lose more slowly than women. The object of this course is weight loss through control of behaviors. Ultimately, the important thing is the behavior change. It takes time, and not everyone learns or responds at the same rate.

If you want to keep a daily record of your weight, choose a standard time each day, preferably post voiding with no clothes on. It is important to weigh at the same time each day because your body weight will fluctuate as much as five or ten pounds during the day. You will also have day-to-day changes in your weight (predominantly from water retention, often related to the salt content of your diet; or, in women, because of your menstrual periods), so don't place too much value on individual highs and lows on the scales.

Starting with Lesson Three, you will be given an average weight loss for the group as a part of each lesson. This will allow you to judge your own weight loss in comparison with that of the entire group. You will be asked to graph your weight loss and the group weight loss on your Master Data Sheet. If you have had no experience with graphs, or do not understand how to do this particular one (at the Third Week), ask your leader. He or she is with you to help you and to teach you to eat differently.

The program consists of ten class lessons spread over 20 weeks. Ten weeks will be used for lessons and ten for practice ("Maintenance"). Each lesson will require one and a half to two hours, including the weigh-in period.

It is very important that by the time the 20 weeks have passed you feel confident that you have mastered all of the techniques in the manual and feel fully able to incorporate them into your daily routine. The watchword during the Maintenance periods will be practice, practice, practice! It is the only way to establish the new behaviors as habits.

Each week the leader will present a lesson which you can follow on the weekly outline. It will be presented very much like a class, with a great deal of discussion from the group. You are urged to take part in the discussion and, if anything is not clear to you, to raise your hand and ask questions. Although some of the material seems repetitious, it is necessary to go over it and over it. What we are aiming for in behavior change is "over-learning." Again, you must learn these behaviors so well that they become habit.

At the end of each lesson, the group leader will go over the homework and explain it in detail. Each set of homework exercises is designed to be successfully completed by the next meeting. Everyone should leave each group session knowing exactly what to do the following week.

People who fail in this program usually pick and choose their techniques. From the outset you must be willing to try all the techniques, ready to give the program a chance to work. Remember, weight loss will be slow, about one pound per week on the average. This will be a process of changing one small behavior at a time, until an entire eating pattern is different.

The majority of the techniques introduced in the first five lessons are designed to eliminate impulse eating, and this will result in weight loss in most people. The second five lessons continue to work on impulse eating. They are also designed to help you increase your exercise, and gain added control over your environment. Eventually, it is your social environment, the people around you, who will help you in your weight control program.

What we want to teach you is more than a way of eating, it is a new way of life. We want to establish habits and ensure that they will last. You don't want to spend a lot of time and money establishing these new patterns and not maximize every chance to ensure that they are permanent.

Our goal in this program is to make you an autonomous weight control therapist. At the termination of the group program, we would like you to feel confident that you can control your eating behaviors. In the years to come you will be able to turn back to this manual anytime you feel out of control, to choose the appropriate techniques to work on, and reinstitute your behavior changes.

Occasionally, the program may seem deceptively simple. At other times, it may seem hopelessly complex. It has been written to provide a variety of techniques, and each person will react to a given technique differently. If you find that any of the techniques are too easy for you, don't withdraw or feel the group is not worth your while. Tell other people how you are able to be successful. Later in the program they may be able to help you with one or two techniques that are easy for them but difficult for you.

Behavior change is a process of taking successive small steps in a consistent direction. In this program, we will take many steps together. Though each is small, they can take you a long way.

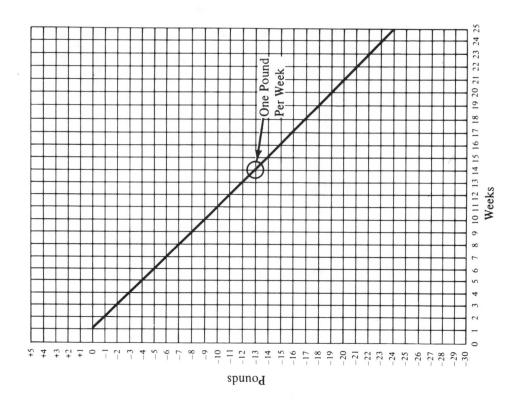

One Pound Per Week

Weeks

Pounds

MASTER DATA SHEET

Name _____

Date _____

Height _____

Date	Weight	Weight Change	Total Wt. Change	Av. Gr. Loss

MASTER DATA SHEET

Name _____

Date _____

Height _____

Date	Weight	Weight Change	Total Wt. Change	Av. Gr. Loss

Group Leader's Copy

Fill in your name, height, weight today, and the date. Give this copy of the Master Data Sheet to your group leader for his records.

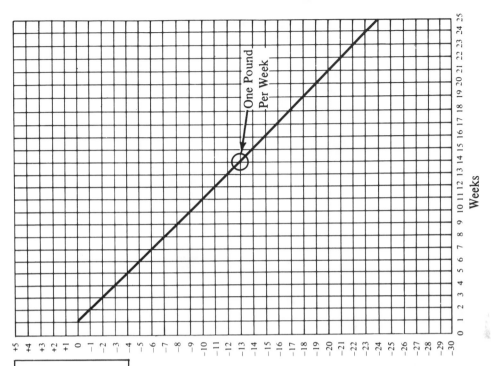

One Pound Per Week

Weeks

Pounds

HOMEWORK CREDIT

Name_____

Lesson	Homework	Refund	Checked by
I. INTRODUCTION TO THE BEHAVIORAL CONTROL OF WEIGHT.			
	A. Week 1 Food Diary	1.00	
	B. House Plan	1.00	
II. CUE ELIMINATION			
	A. Week 2 Food Diary	1.50	
	B. Eating Place Record	1.50	
III. CHANGING THE ACT OF EATING			
	A. Week 3 Food Diary	1.00	
	B. Eating Place Record	.50	
	C. Eating Ratio Column Completed	1.00	
IV. BEHAVIOR CHAINS AND ALTERNATE ACTIVITIES			
	A. Week 4 Food Diary	.50	
	B. Alternate Activities Specified	.50	
	C. Activity Substitutions Recorded	.50	
	D. One Behavior Chain Defined	.50	
	E. Alternate Link for the Behavior Chain	.50	
V. PROBLEM SOLVING			
	A. Week 5 Food Diary	.50	
	B. Daily Behavior Checklist	.50	
	C. Eating Place Record	.50	
	D. Eating Ratio Column Completed	.50	
	E. Behavioral Prescription Sheet	.50	
(Maintenance Period):			
M-1	Maintenance Week 1 Food Diary Maintenance Week 1 Behavior Checklist	0.00	
M-2	Maintenance Week 2 Food Diary Maintenance Week 2 Behavior Checklist	0.00	
M-3	Maintenance Week 3 Food Diary Maintenance Week 3 Behavior Checklist	0.00	
M-4	Maintenance Week 4 Food Diary Maintenance Week 4 Behavior Check List	0.00	
M-5	Maintenance Week 5 Food Diary Maintenance Week 5 Behavior Checklist Behavioral Analysis Form (Week 6 and Week 16)	0.00	

HOMEWORK CREDIT

Name _____ _____

Lesson	Homework	Refund	Checked by
VI. PRE-PLANNING			
	A. Week 6 Food Diary	0.50	
	B. Week 6 Behavior Checklist	1.00	
	C. Pre-planning	1.00	
	D. Behavioral Prescription Sheet	0.50	
VII. CUE ELIMINATION, PART TWO. ENERGY, PART ONE			
	A. Week 7 Food Diary	0.50	
	B. Week 7 Behavior Checklist	0.50	
	C. Pre-planning	1.00	
	D. Minutes of Exercise by Category and Miles Walked Recorded Daily on the Activity Sheet	1.00	
VIII. ENERGY USE, PART TWO			
	A. Week 8 Food Diary	0.50	
	B. Maintenance Behavior Checklist	1.00	
	C. Daily Activity Sheet	1.00	
	D. Daily Energy-Out (activity) Graph	1.00	
IX. SNACKS, CUES AND HOLIDAYS			
	A. Daily Activity Sheet	1.00	
	B. Snack Worksheet	1.00	
	C. Maintenance Behavior Checklist	1.00	
	D. Food Diary (Optional)	–	
X. ENVIRONMENTAL SUPPORT – FAMILY AND FRIENDS			
	A. Maintenance Behavior Checklist	–	
	B. Food Diary (Optional)	–	
	C. Refund – Total (may be returned at the end of the Final Maintenance Period)	–	

Lesson One
INTRODUCTION TO THE BEHAVIORAL CONTROL OF WEIGHT– HABIT AWARENESS

1

Lesson One
INTRODUCTION TO THE BEHAVIORAL
CONTROL OF WEIGHT—HABIT AWARENESS

I. Weigh-in and Distribution of Manuals.

   A. At the beginning of each lesson individual weights will be recorded on the Master Data Sheet.

   B. The manual contains your materials for a 10-lesson course.

      1. Bring the manual with you every meeting.

      2. Each week we will review and discuss the outline of the week's lesson.

      3. Take notes on the outline so that you can review and teach the material during the week, or in the future.

   C. The homework for the first week is the Food Diary and the House Plan. Each week you will receive additional homework forms.

II. Methods of Weight Control.

   A. Weight control programs have traditionally involved diets, drugs, HCG shots (with a 500-calorie diet), hypnosis, psychotherapy, and surgery.

   B. Most of these programs are not effective in the long run because they are time limited. When the program is over, most people resume their old patterns of eating and regain the weight. Nothing has been learned.

   C. This program is aimed at weight loss, but specifically, weight loss as a result of behavior change.

III. Theories of Obesity.

   A. There are many theories why people become obese. Some of the factors which might be involved are genetic, cellular, and endocrine defects, deep-seated psychological problems, family eating patterns, and childhood feeding patterns.

   B. Specific causes can be assigned to less than one percent of all weight problems. (Nevertheless, overweight individuals should have regular checkups with their physicians.)

   C. Regardless of predisposing factors, overweight is a direct result of more energy taken in than burned up. If this imbalance is corrected by changing eating and activity habits, overweight can be overcome.

IV. The Behavioral Model of Weight Control.

    A. Over-eating and inactivity are habits.

    B. If you are overweight because of a learned habit, the solution is to learn new eating behaviors or habits.

    C. This is best done by rearranging your environment so that new habits are more likely to occur than old ones.

    D. In this program the main focus will be to increase the strength of appropriate eating skills rather than trying directly to weaken inappropriate ones.

    E. Changing long-standing habits is difficult. The way to succeed is to make changes, a small step at a time, and to practice each step until it seems like second nature.

    F. Weight reduction is successful only if it lasts indefinitely. Losing weight does not have to be a painful or even a very hungry experience.

    G. To make this program work, behavior change and weight reduction must be high on your list of priorities.

    H. In behavior modification programs, measurement is extremely important. In this program we emphasize habit awareness: observing and keeping records of all your eating behaviors.

V. Assignment: Food Diary and House Plan—Habit Awareness.

    A. The first daily measure we want you to keep is the Food Diary.

        1. The purpose of the Diary is to make you aware of your eating behaviors and to gather baseline information about your eating habits.

        2. The natural tendency when people start to keep a Food Diary is to decrease the amount they eat and to be more selective about their snacks and impulse eating. This is the beginning of behavioral control of your eating habits.

    B. Fill out your Diary according to the enclosed sheet of instructions.

        1. Make the entries immediately after eating.

        2. Don't let the records become inaccurate during over-eating. These are the behaviors which need to be the most accurately recorded.

        3. Save your completed Food Diaries for use in future lessons.

C.   The second part of this week's assignment is the House Plan. This will give you a picture of how spread out or varied your eating habits are at home.

    1.   Draw a simple plan of your house. Label all of the places where food is stored; for example, food in the kitchen, candy on the TV set, crackers by the bed.

    2.   Using the "Location" column on your Food Diary, mark on the House Plan all the places where you ate during the week. Use an "M" to indicate meals and an "S" to indicate where you ate the snacks.

D.   To increase the probability of success in the program, go home and teach each week's lesson to someone else, someone in your family, at school, or at work. This will help them understand what you are doing in this program and will give you a chance to consolidate your learning by teaching someone else.

E.   Next week, the group leader will go over your completed homework when you are weighed. At that time, your Homework Credit schedule will be initialled to indicate which items you completed during the week. The amount of money refunded will be determined by homework completed, not by neatness, spelling, or quality of record-keeping. We do not care if you spill tomato soup or peanut butter on the forms. They are for your use wherever you are.

INSTRUCTIONS FOR FILLING OUT THE FOOD DIARY — Week One

Time: starting time for a meal or snack.

Minutes spent eating: length of the eating episode in minutes.

M/S: meal or snack: indicate type of eating by the appropriate letter, "M" or "S".

H: hunger on a scale of 0 to 3.   0 = no hunger, 3 = extreme hunger

Body position: 1 — walking
                      2 — standing
                      3 — sitting
                      4 — lying down

Activity while eating: Record any activity you carry out while eating, such as watching television, reading, or sweeping the floor.

Location of eating: Record each place you eat; for example your car, kitchen table, or living room couch.

Food type and quantity: Indicate the content of your meal or snack by kind of food and quantity. Choose units of measurement that you will be able to reproduce from week to week. Accuracy is not as important as consistency.

Eating with whom: Indicate with whom you are eating, or if you are eating that meal or snack alone.

Feelings before and during eating: Record your feelings or mood immediately before or during eating. Typical feelings are angry, bored, confused, depressed, frustrated, sad, etc. Many times you will have no feelings associated with eating. In this case, write down "none".

FOOD DIARY – Lesson One

Day of Week _____   Name_____

Time	Minutes Spent Eating	M/S	H	Body Position	Activity While Eating	Location Of Eating	Food Type and Quantity	Eating With Whom	Feeling While Eating
6:00									
11:00									
4:00									
9:00									

M/S: Meal or Snack H: Degree of Hunger (0 = None, 3 = Maximum)
Body Position: 1 = Walking, 2 = Standing, 3 = Sitting, 4 = Lying Down

FOOD DIARY – Lesson One

Day of Week _____   Name_____

Time	Minutes Spent Eating	M/S	H	Body Position	Activity While Eating	Location Of Eating	Food Type and Quantity	Eating With Whom	Feeling While Eating
6:00									
11:00									
4:00									
9:00									

M/S: Meal or Snack H: Degree of Hunger (0 = None, 3 = Maximum)
Body Position: 1 = Walking, 2 = Standing, 3 = Sitting, 4 = Lying Down

FOOD DIARY – Lesson One

Day of Week _____   Name_____

Time	Minutes Spent Eating	M/S	H	Body Position	Activity While Eating	Location Of Eating	Food Type and Quantity	Eating With Whom	Feeling While Eating
6:00									
11:00									
4:00									
9:00									

M/S: Meal or Snack H: Degree of Hunger (0 = None, 3 = Maximum)
Body Position: 1 = Walking, 2 = Standing, 3 = Sitting, 4 = Lying Down

FOOD DIARY – Lesson One

Day of Week _____   Name_____

Time	Minutes Spent Eating	M/S	H	Body Position	Activity While Eating	Location Of Eating	Food Type and Quantity	Eating With Whom	Feeling While Eating
6:00									
11:00									
4:00									
9:00									

M/S: Meal or Snack H: Degree of Hunger (0 = None, 3 = Maximum)
Body Position: 1 = Walking, 2 = Standing, 3 = Sitting, 4 = Lying Down

FOOD DIARY — Lesson One

Day of Week _____   Name_____

Time	Minutes Spent Eating	M/S	H	Body Position	Activity While Eating	Location Of Eating	Food Type and Quantity	Eating With Whom	Feeling While Eating
6:00									
11:00									
4:00									
9:00									

M/S: Meal or Snack H: Degree of Hunger (0 = None, 3 = Maximum)
Body Position: 1 = Walking, 2 = Standing, 3 = Sitting, 4 = Lying Down

1-10

FOOD DIARY – Lesson One

Day of Week _____   Name_____

Time	Minutes Spent Eating	M/S	H	Body Position	Activity While Eating	Location Of Eating	Food Type and Quantity	Eating With Whom	Feeling While Eating
6:00									
11:00									
4:00									
9:00									

M/S: Meal or Snack H: Degree of Hunger (0 = None, 3 = Maximum)
Body Position: 1 = Walking, 2 = Standing, 3 = Sitting, 4 = Lying Down

1-11

FOOD DIARY – Lesson One

Day of Week _____   Name _____

Time	Minutes Spent Eating	M/S	H	Body Position	Activity While Eating	Location Of Eating	Food Type and Quantity	Eating With Whom	Feeling While Eating
6:00									
11:00									
4:00									
9:00									

M/S: Meal or Snack H: Degree of Hunger (0 = None, 3 = Maximum)
Body Position: 1 = Walking, 2 = Standing, 3 = Sitting, 4 = Lying Down

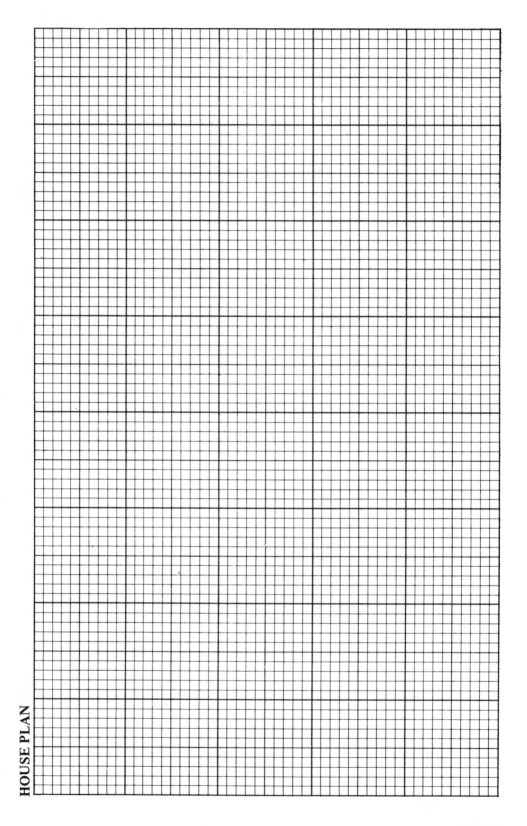

HOUSE PLAN

Lesson Two
CUE ELIMINATION

2

Lesson Two
CUE ELIMINATION

I.   Weigh-in and Homework.

    A.   Record your weight on your Master Data Sheet. Calculate your weight change since last week and put that figure in the columns labeled "Weight Change" and "Total Weight Change."

    B.   Check homework.

        1.   Lesson One Food Diary.

        2.   House Plan.

    C.   The materials for Lesson Two include:

        1.   Lesson Two Outline.

        2.   Lesson Two Food Diary.

        3.   Eating Place Record.

II.   Review.

    A.   Behavioral weight control programs make the assumption that eating, like other behavior, is learned. Our objective in this program is to change your eating behaviors, and to help you lose weight as a result of this change.

    B.   Behavior therapies are based on observation. Your Food Diary will be your chief source of information during the course. Usually, writing down all food intake and related activities exposes patterns of behavior that are not obvious at first.

    C.   To be most effective, the Food Diary should be filled out immediately after each meal. If necessary, record your food intake and the associated information on a "3 x 5" card, or in a small notebook you can carry with you.

III. New Topic: Cue Elimination

    A.   Overweight people are often more sensitive than thin people to external stimuli or cues that trigger eating behaviors.

    B.   One famous psychology experiment demonstrated the powerful effect of perceived time on hunger and showed how much more powerful this was in overweight individuals than in thin subjects.

C. The cues that can evoke the sensation of hunger are almost limitless. They include the time of day, place of eating, and activities associated with eating. Any object in your environment, if paired long enough with eating, will acquire the ability to make you feel hungry.

D. Your House Plan indicates the distribution of your eating behaviors at home. It is common to eat or snack in many places. However, this develops an association between eating and many environmental objects that become food cues.

IV. Cue Elimination: How to Do It:

If you frequently eat in many places, or engage in unassociated activities while eating, you have probably become conditioned to feeling hunger in many situations when your body is not physically hungry. Today's exercise is designed to systematically eliminate some of the environmental or situational controls over your eating.

A. Designate an appropriate eating place at home and for all other places where you normally eat. The designated eating areas may be the kitchen table for breakfast, a restaurant table for lunch, and the dining room table for dinner. Where you designate depends on your individual life style. It should be a place where you can sit down and enjoy your food. Once the eating place is defined, eat all of your meals and snacks at this designated place.

B. Change your habitual eating place at the table. A change in viewpoint often breaks up many old eating habits.

C. When you are eating, only eat. Do not watch television, read, or engage in any activity that is inappropriate to a fine meal. Even arguing during a meal can be a cue for increased eating. You can talk, think, listen to music, or best of all, enjoy your food. Learn to be more of a gourmet: really taste, smell, and experience each mouthful.

D. Try to keep junk foods at a minimum, out of sight or hard to reach.

E. Reduce visual cues. Keep impulse foods in opaque containers. Remove food from all places in the house other than appropriate food storage areas.

F. Do not keep serving containers on the table, or put them at the other end of the table.

V. Feedback.

A. Eliminating strong cues to eat and breaking-up long-standing patterns of eating behavior is a gradual process.

B.   Continuous evaluation or feedback is necessary for you to be able to see how well your behaviors are changing, and to assess your progress. To obtain feedback, you need a visual or graphic record of your behavior. With this type of record, you are immediately aware of changes in your behavior pattern.

C.   Plot your eating places on the enclosed Eating Place Record. The closer you come to a straight line on this diagram, the closer you are to eliminating environmentally cued eating.

D.   Compliment yourself for improved habits. You may feel bad or guilty if old eating behaviors occasionally reappear, but remember, we are looking for improvement, not perfection.

VI.   Homework.

A.   Lesson Two Food Diary.

B.   Eating Place Record filled in for each meal and snack during the coming week.

C.   Designate an appropriate eating place at home and work. Eat all of your meals and snacks at this place.

D.   Change your habitual eating place at the table.

E.   When eating, only eat. No other activities.

F.   Remove food from all places in the house which are not appropriate storage areas.

G.   Keep junk foods out of sight, hidden, hard to get, or don't buy them.

H.   Reduce visual cues for eating. Store food in opaque containers. Remove serving dishes from the table or put them at the opposite end of the table. Mark the last column of the Food Diary "yes" or "no" to indicate whether visual cues were reduced for each meal or snack.

Remember, if you are going to eat, make it worthwhile.

FOOD DIARY – Lesson Two

Day of Week _____   Name _____

Time	Minutes Spent Eating	M/S	H	Activity While Eating	Location of Eating	Type & Quantity of Food	Food Out of Sight
6:00							
11:00							
4:00							
9:00							

M/S – Meal or Snack
H – Hunger (0 = None; 3 = Maximum)

2-5

FOOD DIARY – Lesson Two

Day of Week _____   Name _____

Time	Minutes Spent Eating	M/S	H	Activity While Eating	Location of Eating	Type & Quantity of Food	Food Out of Sight
6:00							
11:00							
4:00							
9:00							

M/S – Meal or Snack
H – Hunger (0 = None; 3 = Maximum)

FOOD DIARY — **Lesson Two**

Day of Week _____   Name _____

Time	Minutes Spent Eating	M/S	H	Activity While Eating	Location of Eating	Type & Quantity of Food	Food Out of Sight
6:00							
11:00							
4:00							
9:00							

M/S — Meal or Snack
H — Hunger (0 = None; 3 = Maximum)

FOOD DIARY – Lesson Two

Day of Week _____   Name _____

Time	Minutes Spent Eating	M/S	H	Activity While Eating	Location of Eating	Type & Quantity of Food	Food Out of Sight
6:00							
11:00							
4:00							
9:00							

M/S – Meal or Snack
H – Hunger (0 = None; 3 = Maximum)

FOOD DIARY – Lesson Two

Day of Week _____   Name _____

Time	Minutes Spent Eating	M/S	H	Activity While Eating	Location of Eating	Type & Quantity of Food	Food Out of Sight
6:00							
11:00							
4:00							
9:00							

M/S – Meal or Snack
H – Hunger (0 = None; 3 = Maximum)

FOOD DIARY — Lesson Two

Day of Week _____   Name _____

Time	Minutes Spent Eating	M/S	H	Activity While Eating	Location of Eating	Type & Quantity of Food	Food Out of Sight
6:00							
11:00							
4:00							
9:00							

M/S — Meal or Snack
H — Hunger (0 = None; 3 = Maximum)

FOOD DIARY – Lesson Two

Day of Week _____   Name _____

Time	Minutes Spent Eating	M/S	H	Activity While Eating	Location of Eating	Type & Quantity of Food	Food Out of Sight
6:00							
11:00							
4:00							
9:00							

M/S – Meal or Snack
H – Hunger (0 = None; 3 = Maximum)

EATING PLACE RECORD

Name _____

(Numbers under the days of the week refer to consecutive eating episodes)

WEEK 2

PLACE	Monday 1 2 3 4 5 6	Tuesday 1 2 3 4 5 6	Wednesday 1 2 3 4 5 6	Thursday 1 2 3 4 5 6	Friday 1 2 3 4 5 6	Saturday 1 2 3 4 5 6	Sunday 1 2 3 4 5 6
Car							
Office desk							
Den – TV room							
Living room							
Designated eating place							
Bedroom							
Kitchen (not at table)							
Other							

WEEK 3

PLACE	Monday 1 2 3 4 5 6	Tuesday 1 2 3 4 5 6	Wednesday 1 2 3 4 5 6	Thursday 1 2 3 4 5 6	Friday 1 2 3 4 5 6	Saturday 1 2 3 4 5 6	Sunday 1 2 3 4 5 6
Car							
Office desk							
Den – TV room							
Living room							
Designated eating place							
Bedroom							
Kitchen (not at table)							
Other							

WEEK 4

PLACE	Monday 1 2 3 4 5 6	Tuesday 1 2 3 4 5 6	Wednesday 1 2 3 4 5 6	Thursday 1 2 3 4 5 6	Friday 1 2 3 4 5 6	Saturday 1 2 3 4 5 6	Sunday 1 2 3 4 5 6
Car							
Office desk							
Den – TV room							
Living room							
Designated eating place							
Bedroom							
Kitchen (not at table)							
Other							

Lesson Three
CHANGING THE ACT OF EATING

3

Lesson Three
CHANGING THE ACT OF EATING

I. Weigh-in and Homework.

    A.   Record your weight and weight change on your Master Data Sheet. Calculate your weight change and total weight change. Enter this on your Master Data Sheet in the appropriate columns.

    B.   Beginning this week you will receive the group average weight loss each meeting. Record it in the appropriate box on the Master Data Sheet. The group average weight change for last week was _____. Graph your total weight change on your Master Data Sheet graph.

    C.   Check homework.

        1.   Lesson Two Food Diary.

        2.   "Food out of sight" column on the Food Diary filled in.

        3.   Eating Place Record.

    D.   The materials for Lesson Three include:

        1.   Outline of Lesson Three.

        2.   Lesson Three Food Diary.

II. Review of the Behavioral Model of Weight Control.

    A.   Eating behaviors are largely learned, and to change them you must learn competing, more appropriate behaviors.

    B.   Basic psychology emphasizes that any object or situation which is paired with eating for a long enough time will eventually acquire the ability to elicit hunger or the desire to eat.

    C.   One of the steps in learning to control your eating behaviors is to change or rearrange your environment so that the learned associations do not have a chance to remind you of food.

    D.   Six cue elimination techniques were introduced last week along with an explanation of how each of them would lead to a decrease in externally-controlled or conditioned hunger.

        1.   By switching places at the table with someone else, you gained a whole new perspective of mealtime.

        2.   When eating, only eat. This is a difficult, but very potent technique, and has the effect of freeing you from a hunger response

to such environmental stimuli as television, the morning paper, and the work on your desk.

3. Remove food from non-storage areas in the house. Food itself is one of the strongest cues to eat, and simply making it less visible often has a profound effect on snacking.

4. Make food less visible, by putting it in "see proof" or opaque containers, or even changing the kitchen lightbulb, or by taking the bulb out of your refrigerator. High impulse or "junk foods" should either not be purchased or kept in a place where they cannot reach out and grab your appetite.

5. Do not leave serving dishes on the table at mealtime—or put them as far away as possible.

6. Designate an appropriate eating place for all of your meals and snacks. This will vary with your actual location, but for each social situation there is one place that can be thought of as most appropriate. The Eating Place Record gives you visual feedback about your success in trying to eat all of your meals at a designated appropriate eating area.

III. Maintenance.

A. If you do not keep track of new behaviors, they will fade with time. To become habits, the activities we suggest must be over-learned, which means they must be practiced until they are routine and actually more comfortable than your old habits.

B. To monitor your progress and to see how well you are able to maintain a habit like eating in one place, fill out an evaluation or feedback form like the Eating Place Record each day.

C. Keep filling out Food Diaries after each meal to remind yourself of the food you eat and of the behaviors associated with eating.

D. When we add new behaviors for you to practice, we will introduce a Daily Behavior Checklist so you can systematically keep track of how well you are doing.

IV. New Technique: Changing the Act of Eating.

A. Many overweight people have a habit of eating in almost a continual stream. This is a bad habit for two reasons: it takes time for the food you eat to be absorbed into your system and decrease the hunger you feel, and you do not have time to really enjoy your food.

B. If a delay can be built into the process of eating, both of these problems can be overcome.

C. Many overweight people have a habit of reloading their fork with food before they have finished chewing the previous forkful. If you learn to swallow the food in your mouth before putting more on your fork, you will automatically extend the length of time a meal takes.

D. The best way to learn this behavior is to try systematically to put your utensils down until each bite has been swallowed. Some people can simply begin to put their utensils down after each bite; others need to work up to it.

E. To develop this behavior, start with an observation of how frequently you put your utensils down during a given time, or an entire meal, and compare this with the total number of bites in the same period of time. A five-minute sample is sufficient to determine your ratio of forks down to swallows. Once this is determined, for example, 1:8 (fork down once for every eight bites swallowed), try to reduce it to once in four bites, then once in two bites, and finally, to putting your utensil down after every bite. Record the ratio of putting utensils down to bites in the last column of this week's Food Diary.

F. If putting utensils down after each bite is already a habit, try the additional technique of introducing a two-minute delay between courses in a meal. Use the time to talk, think, or simply rest.

V. Homework.

A. Fill in Lesson Three Food Diary.

B. Fill in the eating ratio column on the Lesson Three Food Diary.

C. Continue to fill in the Eating Place Record every day.

D. Continue to carry out the cue elimination exercises:

1. Eat all of your meals and snacks in a designated appropriate eating area.

2. When you eat, only eat. No other activities.

3. Eliminate visual cues. Remove food from any inappropriate or non-storage area in the house.

4. Make food inconspicuous. Put it in opaque "see proof" containers.

5. Continue to sit at a different place at the table when you eat.

6. Remove serving dishes from the table, or put them as far away as possible from you on the table.

FOOD DIARY – Lesson Three

Day of Week _____   Name _____

Time	Minutes Spent Eating	M/S	H	Activity While Eating	Location of Eating	Food Type & Quantity	Eating Ratio
6:00							
11:00							
4:00							
9:00							

3-5

FOOD DIARY – Lesson Three

Day of Week _____   Name _____

Time	Minutes Spent Eating	M/S	H	Activity While Eating	Location of Eating	Food Type & Quantity	Eating Ratio
6:00							
11:00							
4:00							
9:00							

FOOD DIARY – Lesson Three

Day of Week _____   Name_____

Time	Minutes Spent Eating	M/S	H	Activity While Eating	Location of Eating	Food Type & Quantity	Eating Ratio
6:00							
11:00							
4:00							
9:00							

FOOD DIARY – **Lesson Three**

Day of Week _____   Name_____

Time	Minutes Spent Eating	M/S	H	Activity While Eating	Location of Eating	Food Type & Quantity	Eating Ratio
6:00							
11:00							
4:00							
9:00							

FOOD DIARY – Lesson Three

Day of Week _____   Name_____

Time	Minutes Spent Eating	M/S	H	Activity While Eating	Location of Eating	Food Type & Quantity	Eating Ratio
6:00							
11:00							
4:00							
9:00							

3-9

FOOD DIARY — **Lesson Three**

Day of Week _____   Name_____

Time	Minutes Spent Eating	M/S	H	Activity While Eating	Location of Eating	Food Type & Quantity	Eating Ratio
6:00							
11:00							
4:00							
9:00							

FOOD DIARY – Lesson Three

Day of Week _____   Name _____

Time	Minutes Spent Eating	M/S	H	Activity While Eating	Location of Eating	Food Type & Quantity	Eating Ratio
6:00							
11:00							
4:00							
9:00							

Lesson Four
BEHAVIOR CHAINS AND ALTERNATE ACTIVITIES

4

Lesson Four
BEHAVIOR CHAINS AND
ALTERNATE ACTIVITIES

I. Weigh-in and Homework.

    A. Record your weight on your Master Data Sheet.

    B. The group average weight loss for last week was_____ .

    C. Check homework.

        1. Lesson Three Food Diary.

        2. Eating ratio column filled in every day.

        3. Eating Place Record completed for the past week.

    D. The materials for Lesson Four include:

        1. Outline of Lesson Four.

        2. Lesson Four Food Diary.

        3. Behavioral Analysis Form.

        4. Alternate Activity Sheet.

II. Review.

    A. Self-observation skills. The Food Diary is a self-observation tool which you have used to assess your eating behaviors. It is a powerful technique that can reshape old eating habits and maintain new ones, because it constantly reminds and sensitizes you to all of the food you eat and the behaviors associated with your eating.

    B. Environmental control. Cue elimination techniques are very important.

        1. Any neutral object can become a stimulus for eating if it is consistently paired with food or eating behaviors.

        2. Cue elimination techniques were suggested to disrupt cue or stimulus-controlled eating. The techniques introduced to neutralize cues were:

            a. Switch places at the table.

            b. When eating, only eat.

            c. Make food invisible, use opaque storage containers, and remove food from non-storage areas.

d.   Minimize the attraction of "junk" or empty calorie food.

   e.   Take serving dishes off the table.

   f.   Do all of your eating in a designated appropriate area.

3.   A feedback scatter diagram, the Eating Place Record, was introduced to help you see your progress. As marks on the diagram approach a straight line, you are eating more and more of your meals in your designated appropriate eating place.

C.   Changing the act of eating. Slowing down eating behaviors was an important technique introduced last week.

   1.   Overweight people tend to eat faster than thin people.

   2.   To interrupt this pattern of rapid eating, we asked you to put your utensils down between bites.

   3.   The ratio of the number of times you put your utensils down, to the number of mouthfuls or swallows, provided feedback about this new behavior.

   4.   If you have mastered putting down your utensils between mouthfuls, introduce a further delay by swallowing your food between bites and adding a pause of two minutes at some point in the meal. Use this time to talk, rest, or simply enjoy pleasant thoughts.

III.   New Technique: Behavior Chains and Alternate Activities.

A.   Substitution of alternate activities can often delay or overcome a hunger response. It is a technique that can be used to eliminate a great deal of snacking; it uses "brain power" rather than "will power."

B.   Alternate activities are effective because behaviors usually occur in chains, and it is usually possible to substitute links in a chain. Eating is often at the end of a chain of responses, and is often one of the terminal events. If the chain is broken at any point, the terminal behavior will probably not occur.

C.   An example of a behavioral chain is seen in the links below, starting with the end of an ample dinner, and eventually connecting with eating a piece of cheesecake, feeling guilty, and wanting another piece of cake.

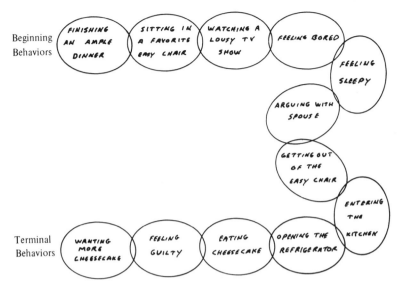

Beginning Behaviors: FINISHING AN AMPLE DINNER → SITTING IN A FAVORITE EASY CHAIR → WATCHING A LOUSY TV SHOW → FEELING BORED → FEELING SLEEPY → ARGUING WITH SPOUSE → GETTING OUT OF THE EASY CHAIR → ENTERING THE KITCHEN → OPENING THE REFRIGERATOR → EATING CHEESECAKE → FEELING GUILTY → WANTING MORE CHEESECAKE: Terminal Behaviors

D. Once the behavior chain has been identified, you can select an alternate activity to substitute for one of the links in the chain. The alternate activity should not lead to eating.

E. To break the behavior chain, choose an alternate activity to fit closely with the link you are replacing. In the above example, you could read a sex book or watch another show when you feel bored. You could take a nap when you feel sleepy, or you could wash the dinner dishes or take a walk before you allowed yourself to open the refrigerator, or you could be prepared with alternate available food for the crisis period.

F. Activities that are appropriate substitutions must be:

1. Readily available.

2. Able to compete with the urge to eat.

3. If possible, incompatible with eating, like a nap.

G. Alternate activity can be:

1. Pleasant activities you have delayed for use as substitutions: hobbies, music, reading, gardening, walking, sports, and sleeping.

2. Necessary activities you have saved to use as substitutions: errands, cleaning, housework, phone calls, bills, washing your hair, taking a bath.

H. Another way to break a behavior chain is to systematically introduce a delay between links in the chain with a timer. Hunger pangs are relatively short-lived and a ten-minute delay may be all you need to prevent an eating episode.

I. Note: A great deal of extra eating is done when people are fatigued, bored, or sad. If you can prevent boredom, or combat it with pre-planned activities, you may be able to prevent over-eating. If you are eating because of simple fatigue, take a ten-minute nap.

IV.   Assignment.

A.   Write down a behavior chain of your own on the Alternate Activity Sheet. Start with the terminal end, eating, and think backward to what behavior or activity immediately preceded eating. Continue working backward as many steps as you can.

B.   Try to introduce a link that leads to a behavior other than eating. Write this substitution down as a side link on your behavior chain.

C.   In class you listed six activities, three pleasant diversions and three necessary activities that can be used to substitute for an eating response. Try to use one each day. Describe the result on your Alternate Activity Sheet.

D.   If you cannot introduce activities into your behavior chains, introduce time. Set a timer for progressively longer periods of time between the urge to snack and the point where you allow yourself to eat.

V.   Homework.

A.   Transfer the information from your Lesson One Food Diary to the places on the Behavioral Analysis Form marked Week One. We will analyze your Lesson Four Food Diary in class next week.

B.   Lesson Four Food Diary.

C.   Eating Ratio filled in every day—try to make it 1:1.

D.   Complete the Eating Place Record.

E.   Write down one of your behavior chains on the Alternate Activity Sheet.

F.   Plan an "unlinking" strategy. Find the weak link in the chain and plan an alternate activity for that weak link.

G.   Substitute an activity from your list of alternate activities for an inappropriate eating episode or snack. Record your successes to share with others next week.

FOOD DIARY – Lesson Four

Day of Week_____   Name_____

Time	Min Spent Eating	M/S	H	Body Position	Activity While Eating	Location of Eating	Food Type and Quantity	Ratio
6:00								
11:00								
4:00								
9:00								

FOOD DIARY — Lesson Four

Day of Week_____   Name _____

Time	Min Spent Eating	M/S	H	Body Position	Activity While Eating	Location of Eating	Food Type and Quantity	Ratio
6:00								
11:00								
4:00								
9:00								

FOOD DIARY – Lesson Four

Day of Week_____   Name _____

Time	Min Spent Eating	M/S	H	Body Position	Activity While Eating	Location of Eating	Food Type and Quantity	Ratio
6:00								
11:00								
4:00								
9:00								

FOOD DIARY – Lesson Four

Day of Week_____   Name_____

Time	Min Spent Eating	M/S	H	Body Position	Activity While Eating	Location of Eating	Food Type and Quantity	Ratio
6:00								
11:00								
4:00								
9:00								

FOOD DIARY – Lesson Four

Day of Week_____   Name_____

Time	Min Spent Eating	M/S	H	Body Position	Activity While Eating	Location of Eating	Food Type and Quantity	Ratio
6:00								
11:00								
4:00								
9:00								

FOOD DIARY – Lesson Four

Day of Week_____   Name_____

Time	Min Spent Eating	M/S	H	Body Position	Activity While Eating	Location of Eating	Food Type and Quantity	Ratio
6:00								
11:00								
4:00								
9:00								

4-11

FOOD DIARY – Lesson Four

Day of Week_____   Name_____

Time	Min Spent Eating	M/S	H	Body Position	Activity While Eating	Location of Eating	Food Type and Quantity	Ratio
6:00								
11:00								
4:00								
9:00								

BEHAVIORAL ANALYSIS FORM
TIME OF EATING

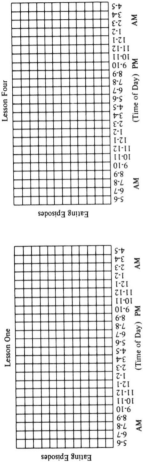

Lesson One

Eating Episodes

5-6 6-7 7-8 8-9 9-10 10-11 11-12 12-1 1-2 2-3 3-4 4-5 5-6 6-7 7-8 8-9 9-10 10-11 11-12 12-1 1-2 2-3 3-4 4-5
AM   (Time of Day) PM   AM

Lesson Four

Eating Episodes

5-6 6-7 7-8 8-9 9-10 10-11 11-12 12-1 1-2 2-3 3-4 4-5 5-6 6-7 7-8 8-9 9-10 10-11 11-12 12-1 1-2 2-3 3-4 4-5
AM   (Time of Day) PM   AM

Indicate the time of day for each eating episode during the week by making a mark in the square above the appropriate time of day. Start with the bottom row of boxes. If you have a second eating episode during the week within that time range, indicate it by filling in the next box in that column. For example, if you had a snack at 10:30 am, you would fill in the first box in the time of day column labeled "10-11 am." If the next day, you had breakfast at 10:15 am, you would blacken in the next box up in that same column. If that same day, you had a snack at 10:50 am, you would indicate this by marking the third box in the same column. When you have entered an entire week's eating pattern in these boxes, you will have a graph which shows the distribution of your eating during the week.

MINUTES SPENT EATING

	Lesson One		Lesson Four	
	Meal	Snack	Meal	Snack
0-5 minutes.......	____	____	____	____
5-10 minutes.......	____	____	____	____
10-15 minutes......	____	____	____	____
15-20 minutes......	____	____	____	____
20-30 minutes......	____	____	____	____
over 30 minutes.....	____	____	____	____

Indicate the duration of *each* of your eating episodes by making a tally mark on the line under the appropriate heading — "meal" or "snack". For example, if breakfast took seven minutes, put a mark under the word "meal" on the line labeled "5-10 minutes." If you had a mid-afternoon snack that lasted 13 minutes, put a mark under "snack" on the line labeled "10-15 minutes." If you had six meals, each 5-10 minutes long, you would have six talleys (卌 I) in the meal column on the line marked 5-10 minutes.

(Adapted from and used by permission of Leonard S. Levitz, Ph.D., and Henry A. Jordan, M.D., University of Pennsylvania School of Medicine, "Analysis of Food Intake and Energy Expenditure," Copyright, 1973.)

BEHAVIORAL ANALYSIS FORM

DEGREE OF HUNGER

	Lesson One			Lesson Four	
	Meal	Snack		Meal	Snack
0 – none	_____	_____	0 – none	_____	_____
1 – some	_____	_____	1 – some	_____	_____
2 – hungry...	_____	_____	2 – hungry ...	_____	_____
3 – extreme..	_____	_____	3 – extreme ..	_____	_____

Put a tally mark on the appropriate line to indicate the degree of hunger you felt at the beginning of every episode of eating during the week. For example, if you had a snack and were not hungry, put a mark under snack on the line labeled "none." If you felt like you were starving to death when you had dinner, put a mark under "meal" on the line labeled "extreme." (Note: Use the same numbers that appear on your Week One Food Diary.)

BODY POSITION WHILE EATING

	Lesson One			Lesson Four	
	Meal	Snack		Meal	Snack
Walking	_____	_____	Walking	_____	_____
Standing ...	_____	_____	Standing ...	_____	_____
Sitting	_____	_____	Sitting	_____	_____
Lying Down.	_____	_____	Lying Down.	_____	_____

Put a tally mark on the appropriate line to indicate your body position during each episode of eating for the week. For example, if you had a snack while walking around the grocery store, put a mark under "snack" on the line labeled "walking". If you ate dinner lying in bed watching television, put a mark under "meal" on the line labeled "lying down."

ACTIVITIES WHILE EATING

	Lesson One		Lesson Four	
	Meal	Snack	Meal	Snack
None: only eating	_____	_____	_____	_____
Talking...............	_____	_____	_____	_____
Listening to music or radio.....	_____	_____	_____	_____
Reading a book or paper......	_____	_____	_____	_____
Watching television..........	_____	_____	_____	_____
Cooking-working in kitchen	_____	_____	_____	_____
Working-studying...........	_____	_____	_____	_____
Other	_____	_____	_____	_____

Put a tally mark on the appropriate line to indicate activities that are associated with your episodes of eating. For example, if you ate lunch while working at your desk, put a mark under "meal" on the line labeled "working." If you had a snack while preparing dinner, put a mark under the "snack" column on the line labeled "cooking."

(Adapted from and used by permission of Leonard S. Levitz, Ph.D., and Henry A. Jordan, M.D., University of Pennsylvania School of Medicine, "Analysis of Food Intake and Energy Expenditure," Copyright, 1973.)

ALTERNATE ACTIVITY SHEET

SUBSTITUTE ACTIVITIES

Pleasant Activities   1. _____

2. _____

3. _____

Necessary Activities   1. _____

2. _____

3. _____

Situations when used   1. _____

2. _____

3. _____

4. _____

5. _____

6. _____

7. _____

BEHAVIOR CHAIN

Identify the links in your eating response chain on the following diagram. Draw a line through the chain where it was interrupted. Add the link you substituted and the new chain of behaviors this substitution started.

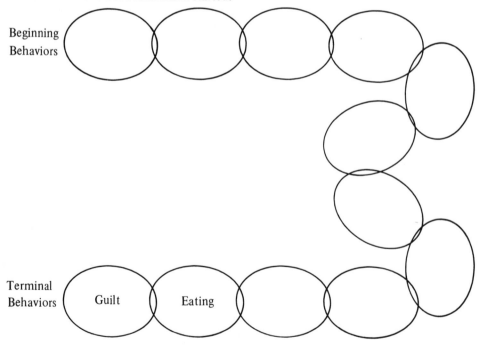

Lesson Five
BEHAVIORAL ANALYSIS, PROGRESS, AND PROBLEM SOLVING

5

Lesson Five
BEHAVIORAL ANALYSIS,
PROGRESS, AND PROBLEM SOLVING

I.   Weigh-In and Homework.

    A.   Record your weight on the Master Data Sheet.

    B.   The group average weight loss for last week was_____ .

    C.   Check homework.

        1.   Lesson Four Food Diary.

        2.   Eating ratio column filled out for each day.

        3.   Eating Place Record completed.

        4.   One behavior chain defined on the Alternate Activity Sheet.

        5.   At least four alternate activities listed on the Alternate Activity Sheet.

        6.   Alternate activity substitutions recorded on the Alternate Activity Sheet.

        7.   Behavioral Analysis Form filled in with data from Lesson One Food Diary.

    D.   The materials for Lesson Five include:

        1.   Outline of Lesson Five.

        2.   Lesson Five Food Diary and Diaries for Maintenance Weeks 1-5.

        3.   Behavioral Prescription Sheet.

        4.   Daily Behavior Checklist for Maintenance Weeks 1-5.

II. Review.

    A.   A Food Diary gives you immediate information about the way you eat and the content of your meals.

    B.   The Eating Place Record is a scatter diagram which shows your progress toward the goal of eating at your designated eating places. Restricting your eating to such appropriate places neutralizes many environmental cues that make you feel hungry when you do not need food.

    C.   The Eating Ratio is a way of measuring a change you introduced in one of your basic eating behaviors. Putting your utensils down between bites has allowed you to stretch a meal out over a longer period of time, to enjoy it more, and to eat less food.

    D.   Behavior Chains. Behaviors tend to occur in chains. The occurrence of a behavior in the chain makes the occurrence of the next behavior more probable.

        1.   Sometimes behavior chains can be most easily identified by working from the terminal end backwards, e.g., eating cheesecake may be ultimately preceded by leaving the dinner table to watch a dull television program.

        2.   Often it is possible to substitute an alternate activity for one of the links of the chain. When this happens, the chain usually is broken and the activity does not occur.

        3.   The earlier in the chain the break is made, the easier it is to introduce an alternate activity.

        4.   When you have only the terminal end of the chain to manipulate, the introduction of a time delay, or a behavior incompatible with eating is often effective.

III.   New Technique: Problem Solving or Becoming Your Own Therapist.

    A.   During the first three weeks, we have defined problem behaviors and created solutions for you. The problems we have worked with to date are shared by almost everyone with a weight problem.

    B.   This week we want you to begin to solve behavioral problems that are uniquely yours. We want you to start becoming your own behavior therapist. Problem-solving skills will enable you to deal with any maladaptive or problem behaviors that arise once this course is over.

    C.   We have arbitrarily divided the problem solving into five steps:

        1.   <u>Observation and long-term goal definition</u>. The Food Diary is an example of observation; the long-term goal is losing weight.

        2.   <u>Definition of specific problems or short-term goal setting.</u> Break the problem into small steps, each of which can be specifically defined and approached with a reasonable chance of success.

        3.   <u>Create alternative plans to solve the specific problem you have defined</u>. BRAINSTORM—uncritically think of as many solutions to the problem as you can. Write them all down.

        4.   <u>Decision-making, or choosing the most appropriate plan</u>. Choose a plan that looks like it will solve your problem, that has a good

chance of success, but still takes into consideration factors such as pleasure and your life style.

5. <u>Evaluation and feedback</u>. If you don't know where you are, you will never know where you are going. Keep evaluating your progress.

IV. Practice Problem-solving Techniques.

A. To evaluate your progress and define specific problems, we would like you to complete your Behavioral Analysis Form with information from your Lesson One and Four Food Diaries. The easiest way to do this is to work with another group member. Have your partner read off the items from the Diary sheets while you mark the appropriate sections of your Behavioral Analysis Form.

B. Compare the analysis patterns for Week One and Week Four. You should be proud of the positive changes you see in your eating behaviors. These behaviors are hard to change. Often people are not aware of the magnitude of their change until they see it on paper.

C. The Eating Place Record should be considered part of the analysis form. It indicates the change in your eating place over the past three weeks.

D. Based on the information in your partner's Food Diary and Behavioral Analysis Form, define a very specific problem for him to work on for the next week. Record it on the Behavioral Prescription Sheet. This can include items on the analysis form, like eating when he is not hungry. It can also be a problem discovered in the Food Diary, like eating a whole pizza each weekend night.

E. Make a list of possible solutions and discuss the alternatives with your partner.

F. Choose the best plan or solution for the defined problem together.

G. Devise a technique of monitoring behaviors or giving feedback about progress towards the goal you have set up. The blank columns on the Food Diary can be used for this purpose.

H. After you have been the therapist for your partner, reverse roles and have him help you with the same project.

I. By the end of the lesson today each member should have a Behavioral Prescription Sheet completely filled out. During the coming weeks, try to solve the defined problem by the method you have designated. If you find this problem is easily solved, choose another—begin to use your talents as a behavior therapist.

V. Maintenance.

    A. The Daily Behavior Checklist is a way of keeping track of all the behaviors we have covered in the past five weeks.

        1. Read the Daily Behavior Checklist each morning before breakfast to remind yourself of your new eating behaviors. Tape the checklist to the bathroom mirror if necessary.

        2. Rate yourself each evening after dinner on how well you carried out the listed behaviors during the day. Use a scale of 1-3, with 3 indicating the greatest success.

    B. Although the weekly check-in meetings are optional, we highly recommend that you attend as many as possible. This five-week period is to give you time to practice what you have learned in the first five lessons. Included in today's packet of materials are Food Diaries and Daily Behavior Checklists for the coming weeks. We will not check them unless you ask. Keeping track of your own behaviors is part of behavior Maintenance.

    C. When we resume regular meetings in five weeks, we will go over the Behavior Checklists with you and assess how well you have maintained your behavior changes.

VI. Homework.

    A. Lesson Five Food Diary (and Diaries for Maintenance Weeks 1-5).

    B. Lesson Five Daily Behavior Checklist (and Checklists for Maintenance Weeks 1-5).

    C. Problem solving. Solve at least the problem defined on the Behavior Prescription Sheet. Use the blank columns of the Food Diary for individual problems you develop during the five-week break

    D. Master Data Sheet. Plot your weekly weight change. If necessary, arrange an individual time each week to be weighed.

    E. Maintenance: PRACTICE, PRACTICE, PRACTICE!

FOOD DIARY – Lesson Five,

Day of Week:_____   Name_____

Time	M/S	H	Food Type and Quantity	Eating Ratio
6:00				
11:00				
4:00				
9:00				

FOOD DIARY – Lesson Five,

Day of Week:_____   Name_____

Time	M/S	H	Food Type and Quantity	Eating Ratio
6:00				
11:00				
4:00				
9:00				

FOOD DIARY – **Lesson Five,**

Day of Week:_____   Name_____

Time	M/S	H	Food Type and Quantity	Eating Ratio
6:00				
11:00				
4:00				
9:00				

FOOD DIARY — Lesson Five,

Day of Week:_____   Name_____

Time	M/S	H	Food Type and Quantity	Eating Ratio
6:00				
11:00				
4:00				
9:00				

FOOD DIARY – Lesson Five,

Day of Week:_____   Name_____

Time	M/S	H	Food Type and Quantity	Eating Ratio
6:00				
11:00				
4:00				
9:00				

FOOD DIARY — Lesson Five,

Day of Week:_____   Name_____

Time	M/S	H	Food Type and Quantity	Eating Ratio
6:00				
11:00				
4:00				
9:00				

FOOD DIARY – Lesson Five,

Day of Week:_____   Name_____

Time	M/S	H	Food Type and Quantity	Eating Ratio
6:00				
11:00				
4:00				
9:00				

DAILY BEHAVIOR CHECKLIST — Lesson Five,

Points: Most of the time, or yes = 3
Sometimes   = 2
Not at all, or no   = 1

Days of the Week

	1	2	3	4	5	6	7
1. *Daily Checklist* a. Morning review (3 if I read the checklist)							
b. Evening scoring (3 if I rated myself)							
2. *Food Diary* a. Recording my food							
3. *Cue Elimination* a. Designated eating place							
b. Change place at table							
c. Only eating when eating							
d. Reduce visual cues-storage, opaque containers							
e. Serving dishes off the table							
f. Junk food out of sight							
4. *Eating Delay* a. Utensils down between mouthfuls							
b. Swallowing each forkful before adding the next							
c. Chewing slowly and thoroughly							
d. Enjoying the meal							
e. Programming a delay in the meal							
5. *Becoming My Own Therapist* a. Individual problem solving							
DAILY TOTALS							

Total Points For the Week _____   Weight _____

BEHAVIORAL PRESCRIPTION SHEET

Name _____

Partner _____

Problem _____
_____
_____
_____

Solutions_____
_____
_____
_____
_____
_____
_____
_____

Plan _____
_____
_____
_____
_____

Feedback_____
_____
_____

Consultation_____

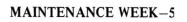

MAINTENANCE WEEK—5

FOOD DIARY – Maintenance Week One

Day of Week:_____   Name_____

Time	M/S	H	Food Type and Quantity	Eating Ratio
6:00				
11:00				
4:00				
9:00				

FOOD DIARY — Maintenance Week One

Day of Week:_____   Name_____

Time	M/S	H	Food Type and Quantity	Eating Ratio
6:00				
11:00				
4:00				
9:00				

M-3

FOOD DIARY — **Maintenance Week One**

Day of Week: _____   Name _____

Time	M/S	H	Food Type and Quantity	Eating Ratio
6:00				
11:00				
4:00				
9:00				

FOOD DIARY — Maintenance Week One

Day of Week:_____   Name_____

Time	M/S	H	Food Type and Quantity	Eating Ratio
6:00				
11:00				
4:00				
9:00				

M-5

FOOD DIARY – Maintenance Week One

Day of Week:_____   Name_____

Time	M/S	H	Food Type and Quantity	Eating Ratio
6:00				
11:00				
4:00				
9:00				

M-6

FOOD DIARY – Maintenance Week One

Day of Week: _____   Name _____

Time	M/S	H	Food Type and Quantity	Eating Ratio
6:00				
11:00				
4:00				
9:00				

M-7

FOOD DIARY – Maintenance Week One

Day of Week:_____   Name_____

Time	M/S	H	Food Type and Quantity	Eating Ratio
6:00				
11:00				
4:00				
9:00				

DAILY BEHAVIOR CHECKLIST — Maintenance Week One

Points: Most of the time, or yes = 3
         Sometimes   = 2
         Not at all, or no   = 1

	Days of the Week						
	1	2	3	4	5	6	7
1. *Daily Checklist* a. Morning review (3 if I read the checklist)							
b. Evening scoring (3 if I rated myself)							
2. *Food Diary* a. Recording my food							
3. *Cue Elimination* a. Designated eating place							
b. Change place at table							
c. Only eating when eating							
d. Reduce visual cues-storage, opaque containers							
e. Serving dishes off the table							
f. Junk food out of sight							
4. *Eating Delay* a. Utensils down between mouthfuls							
b. Swallowing each forkful before adding the next							
c. Chewing slowly and thoroughly							
d. Enjoying the meal							
e. Programming a delay in the meal							
5. *Becoming My Own Therapist* a. Individual problem solving							
DAILY TOTALS							

Total Points For the Week _____   Weight _____

FOOD DIARY – Maintenance Week Two

Day of Week:_____   Name_____

Time	M/S	H	Food Type and Quantity	Eating Ratio
6:00				
11:00				
4:00				
9:00				

FOOD DIARY – **Maintenance Week Two**

Day of Week:_____   Name_____

Time	M/S	H	Food Type and Quantity	Eating Ratio
6:00				
11:00				
4:00				
9:00				

FOOD DIARY – **Maintenance Week Two**

Day of Week:_____   Name_____

Time	M/S	H	Food Type and Quantity	Eating Ratio
6:00				
11:00				
4:00				
9:00				

FOOD DIARY – **Maintenance Week Two**

Day of Week:_____   Name_____

Time	M/S	H	Food Type and Quantity	Eating Ratio
6:00				
11:00				
4:00				
9:00				

FOOD DIARY — Maintenance Week Two

Day of Week:_____   Name_____

Time	M/S	H	Food Type and Quantity	Eating Ratio
6:00				
11:00				
4:00				
9:00				

FOOD DIARY – Maintenance Week Two

Day of Week:_____   Name_____

Time	M/S	H	Food Type and Quantity	Eating Ratio
6:00				
11:00				
4:00				
9:00				

FOOD DIARY — Maintenance Week Two

Day of Week:_____   Name_____

Time	M/S	H	Food Type and Quantity	Eating Ratio
6:00				
11:00				
4:00				
9:00				

DAILY BEHAVIOR CHECKLIST — Maintenance Week Two

Points: Most of the time, or yes = 3
        Sometimes   = 2
        Not at all, or no   = 1

	Days of the Week						
	1	2	3	4	5	6	7
1. *Daily Checklist* a. Morning review (3 if I read the checklist)							
b. Evening scoring (3 if I rated myself)							
2. *Food Diary* a. Recording my food							
3. *Cue Elimination* a. Designated eating place							
b. Change place at table							
c. Only eating when eating							
d. Reduce visual cues-storage, opaque containers							
e. Serving dishes off the table							
f. Junk food out of sight							
4. *Eating Delay* a. Utensils down between mouthfuls							
b. Swallowing each forkful before adding the next							
c. Chewing slowly and thoroughly							
d. Enjoying the meal							
e. Programming a delay in the meal							
5. *Becoming My Own Therapist* a. Individual problem solving							
DAILY TOTALS							

Total Points For the Week _____   Weight _____

M-17

FOOD DIARY – Maintenance Week Three

Day of Week:_____   Name_____

Time	M/S	H	Food Type and Quantity	Eating Ratio
6:00				
11:00				
4:00				
9:00				

FOOD DIARY – Maintenance Week Three

Day of Week: _____   Name _____

Time	M/S	H	Food Type and Quantity	Eating Ratio
6:00				
11:00				
4:00				
9:00				

FOOD DIARY – **Maintenance Week Three**

Day of Week:_____   Name_____

Time	M/S	H	Food Type and Quantity	Eating Ratio
6:00				
11:00				
4:00				
9:00				

FOOD DIARY – Maintenance Week Three

Day of Week:_____   Name_____

Time	M/S	H	Food Type and Quantity	Eating Ratio
6:00				
11:00				
4:00				
9:00				

FOOD DIARY – Maintenance Week Three

Day of Week: _____   Name _____

Time	M/S	H	Food Type and Quantity	Eating Ratio
6:00				
11:00				
4:00				
9:00				

FOOD DIARY – Maintenance Week Three

Day of Week:_____   Name_____

Time	M/S	H	Food Type and Quantity	Eating Ratio
6:00				
11:00				
4:00				
9:00				

M-23

FOOD DIARY – **Maintenance Week Three**

Day of Week:_____   Name_____

Time	M/S	H	Food Type and Quantity	Eating Ratio
6:00				
11:00				
4:00				
9:00				

DAILY BEHAVIOR CHECKLIST – Maintenance Week Three

Points: Most of the time, or yes = 3
        Sometimes   = 2
        Not at all, or no   = 1

Days of the Week

	1	2	3	4	5	6	7
1. *Daily Checklist* a. Morning review (3 if I read the checklist)							
b. Evening scoring (3 if I rated myself)							
2. *Food Diary* a. Recording my food							
3. *Cue Elimination* a. Designated eating place							
b. Change place at table							
c. Only eating when eating							
d. Reduce visual cues-storage, opaque containers							
e. Serving dishes off the table							
f. Junk food out of sight							
4. *Eating Delay* a. Utensils down between mouthfuls							
b. Swallowing each forkful before adding the next							
c. Chewing slowly and thoroughly							
d. Enjoying the meal							
e. Programming a delay in the meal							
5. *Becoming My Own Therapist* a. Individual problem solving							
DAILY TOTALS							

Total Points For the Week _____   Weight _____

FOOD DIARY – Maintenance Week Four

Day of Week:_____   Name_____

Time	M/S	H	Food Type and Quantity	Eating Ratio
6:00				
11:00				
4:00				
9:00				

FOOD DIARY — Maintenance Week Four

Day of Week:_____   Name_____

Time	M/S	H	Food Type and Quantity	Eating Ratio
6:00				
11:00				
4:00				
9:00				

FOOD DIARY – Maintenance Week Four

Day of Week:_____   Name_____

Time	M/S	H	Food Type and Quantity	Eating Ratio
6:00				
11:00				
4:00				
9:00				

FOOD DIARY — **Maintenance Week Four**

Day of Week:_____   Name_____

Time	M/S	H	Food Type and Quantity	Eating Ratio
6:00				
11:00				
4:00				
9:00				

FOOD DIARY   Maintenance Week Four

Day of Week:_____   Name_____

Time	M/S	H	Food Type and Quantity	Eating Ratio
6:00				
11:00				
4:00				
9:00				

M-30

FOOD DIARY — Maintenance Week Four

Day of Week:_____   Name_____

Time	M/S	H	Food Type and Quantity	Eating Ratio
6:00				
11:00				
4:00				
9:00				

FOOD DIARY – **Maintenance Week Four**

Day of Week:_____   Name_____

Time	M/S	H	Food Type and Quantity	Eating Ratio
6:00				
11:00				
4:00				
9:00				

DAILY BEHAVIOR CHECKLIST – **Maintenance Week Four**

Points: Most of the time, or yes = 3
         Sometimes   = 2
         Not at all, or no   = 1

Days of the Week

	1	2	3	4	5	6	7
1. *Daily Checklist* a. Morning review (3 if I read the checklist)							
b. Evening scoring (3 if I rated myself)							
2. *Food Diary* a. Recording my food							
3. *Cue Elimination* a. Designated eating place							
b. Change place at table							
c. Only eating when eating							
d. Reduce visual cues-storage, opaque containers							
e. Serving dishes off the table							
f. Junk food out of sight							
4. *Eating Delay* a. Utensils down between mouthfuls							
b. Swallowing each forkful before adding the next							
c. Chewing slowly and thoroughly							
d. Enjoying the meal							
e. Programming a delay in the meal							
5. *Becoming My Own Therapist* a. Individual problem solving							
DAILY TOTALS							

Total Points For the Week ——————   Weight ——————

M-33

MAINTENANCE WEEK—5

This is the final week of your Maintenance program. This practice period of five weeks was included in the behavior change program for a specific reason: new behaviors tend to fade away and are forgotten if they are not practiced. During the past month, we have asked you to continue keeping a Food Diary and a Behavior Checklist. We have also stressed the importance of monitoring your eating behaviors daily to give yourself feedback, and to tell yourself how well you are practicing your new eating habits.

For this final Maintenance Week, we want you to keep a complete Food Diary. It is similar to the one you filled out during the fourth week of the course. We will go over it in detail next lesson with a Behavioral Analysis Form, and determine how well you have maintained your new eating skills—and how close they are to becoming habit.

FOOD DIARY – Maintenance Week Five

Day of Week_____   Name_____

Time	Min Spent Eating	M/S	H	Body Position	Activity While Eating	Location of Eating	Food Type and Quantity	Ratio
6:00								
11:00								
4:00								
9:00								

M-35

FOOD DIARY — Maintenance Week Five

Day of Week_____   Name_____

Time	Min Spent Eating	M/S	H	Body Position	Activity While Eating	Location of Eating	Food Type and Quantity	Ratio
6:00								
11:00								
4:00								
9:00								

FOOD DIARY – Maintenance Week Five

Day of Week_____   Name_____

Time	Min Spent Eating	M/S	H	Body Position	Activity While Eating	Location of Eating	Food Type and Quantity	Ratio
6:00								
11:00								
4:00								
9:00								

M-37

FOOD DIARY — Maintenance Week Five

Day of Week_____   Name _____

Time	Min Spent Eating	M/S	H	Body Position	Activity While Eating	Location of Eating	Food Type and Quantity	Ratio
6:00								
11:00								
4:00								
9:00								

M-38

FOOD DIARY – Maintenance Week Five

Day of Week_____   Name_____

Time	Min Spent Eating	M/S	H	Body Position	Activity While Eating	Location of Eating	Food Type and Quantity	Ratio
6:00								
11:00								
4:00								
9:00								

M-39

FOOD DIARY – Maintenance Week Five

Day of Week_____   Name_____

Time	Min Spent Eating	M/S	H	Body Position	Activity While Eating	Location of Eating	Food Type and Quantity	Ratio
6:00								
11:00								
4:00								
9:00								

FOOD DIARY — Maintenance Week Five

Day of Week_____   Name_____

Time	Min Spent Eating	M/S	H	Body Position	Activity While Eating	Location of Eating	Food Type and Quantity	Ratio
6:00								
11:00								
4:00								
9:00								

DAILY BEHAVIOR CHECKLIST — Maintenance Week Five

Points: Most of the time, or yes = 3
        Sometimes   = 2
        Not at all, or no   = 1

Days of the Week

	1	2	3	4	5	6	7
1. *Daily Checklist* a. Morning review (3 if I read the checklist)							
b. Evening scoring (3 if I rated myself)							
2. *Food Diary* a. Recording my food							
3. *Cue Elimination* a. Designated eating place							
b. Change place at table							
c. Only eating when eating							
d. Reduce visual cues-storage, opaque containers							
e. Serving dishes off the table							
f. Junk food out of sight							
4. *Eating Delay* a. Utensils down between mouthfuls							
b. Swallowing each forkful before adding the next							
c. Chewing slowly and thoroughly							
d. Enjoying the meal							
e. Programming a delay in the meal							
5. *Becoming My Own Therapist* a. Individual problem solving							
DAILY TOTALS							

Total Points For the Week _____   Weight _____

Lesson Six
PRE-PLANNING

6

Lesson Six
PRE-PLANNING

I.   Weigh-in.

    A.   Record your weight on your Master Data Sheet.

    B.   The cumulative group average weight loss at Lesson Five was _____.

    C.   The cumulative average weight loss at Maintenance Lesson Five was_____.

    D.   Check homework.

        1.   Behavioral Prescription Sheet—Lesson Five.

        2.   Maintenance Week Five Food Diary.

        3.   Maintenance Week Five Behavior Checklist.

    E.   The materials for Lesson Six include:

        1.   Outline, Lesson Six.

        2.   Lesson Six Food Diary.

        3.   Lesson Six Behavior Checklist.

        4.   Behavioral Prescription Sheet.

        5.   Behavioral Analysis and Feedback Form.

II. Maintenance.

    A.   Maintenance of weight loss is the only objective measure we have of behavior change. We presume weight loss is maintained in proportion to the changes in eating behaviors.

    B.   The five-week Maintenance or practice period you completed today was included in the program to allow you time to consolidate and practice all of the material presented up to this point.

    C.   The Behavior Checklist gives you information about how well you are changing your eating behaviors. The daily ritual of reading the list in the morning before breakfast and checking it off each evening after dinner reminds you of the behaviors you are trying to learn, and keeps track of how well you are maintaining your new eating habits.

    D.   The key to habit change is over-learning. The only way to over-learn is to PRACTICE, PRACTICE, PRACTICE!

III.   Review: Problem Solving.

    A.   Today we are starting the second half of the program. You need to know where you stand, what your successes are, and what you need to review. For Maintenance Week Five, we asked you to fill out a detailed Food Diary. At the end of today's lesson, we want you to go over these Food Diaries with a Behavioral Analysis Form.

    B.   Problem solving was introduced as a general behavioral technique that will continue to be of use when the course is over. We divided problem solving into five parts:

        1.   Observation and long-term goal definition.

        2.   Identification of specific problems.

        3.   Creative problem solving or brainstorming.

        4.   Choosing a plan of action.

        5.   Evaluation and feedback.

    C.   The goal of the problem solving exercise was to train you to spot eating problems, to formulate plans to change these problems, and to evaluate your progress once you have carried out your plan.

    D.   Last lesson you exchanged Food Diaries with another group member. This allowed you to practice with someone else's problems, and gave you the benefit of someone else's ideas. At the end of last lesson we asked all of you to fill out a Behavioral Prescription Sheet for yourself.

    E.   At the end of the lesson today, we will want you to choose a partner again, fill out another Behavioral Analysis Form and work together on problem solving.

IV.   New Technique: Pre-planning What You Eat.

    A.   Pre-planning is a technique that many people find extremely useful and correspondingly difficult. It involves thinking ahead about food and the circumstances of eating.

    B.   Pre-planning is the first step in changing your self-instructions or internal dialogues that determine when, where, and what you eat. As thinking ahead about food becomes a habit, the effect of impulse on eating diminishes.

    C.   Pre-planning can be broken into steps:

        1.   Set aside a time to pre-plan.

2.   Write down your planned menu on your Food Diary—use a different color ink. After the meal you planned, correct your Food Diary.

3.   Plan ahead for restaurants and parties—work out strategies in advance for drinks and high caloric entrees. Use the skills you have learned here to cope with dinner parties, e.g., slow down and enjoy yourself.

4.   Some people find it easier to pre-prepare snacks than to pre-plan them.

D.   Pre-planning what you buy.

A related pre-planning technique applies to shopping for food. Write a shopping list in advance with brand names and quantities. Go to the store on a full stomach and try to buy only the items on your list. Snacks that aren't bought will never be consumed.

E.   Because pre-planning involves a fundamental change in the way you think about food, it should be approached slowly. Insure your success by starting with one meal or snack a day, and increasing the amount of pre-planning when you feel comfortable.

F.   Check off pre-planning on your Behavior Checklist for next week.

V.   Periodic Feedback and Problem Solving.

A.   Periodically it is necessary to analyze your behavior patterns and see how well you are doing with your behavior change program. Although we have built this into the weekly lesson, it is a process that will continue in some form for the years of Maintenance after the course is completed.

B.   Based on your food analysis from last week:

1.   Define a specific problem.

2.   Make a list of as many solutions to the problem as you can—brainstorm.

3.   Pick the best solution.

4.   Devise some form of feedback or self-evaluation so you know whether you are successful in solving the problem.

C.   Periodic practice in problem solving will help you to become your own behavior therapist.

VI.   Homework.

    A.   Lesson Six Food Diary.

    B.   Lesson Six Behavior Checklist.

    C.   Pre-plan one or more meals or snacks each day on your Food Diary. Correct the pre-planned menu after you eat the meal. Use a different color ink for correcting. You will receive immediate feedback through the amount of two-color entries in your Food Diary for the week.

    D.   Complete a Behavioral Prescription Sheet today, and enter your progress with the problem you choose on your Food Diary or another feedback or self-evaluation form.

FOOD DIARY – Lesson Six

Day of Week _____   Name_____

Time	Minutes Spent Eating	M/S	H	Food Type & Quantity	Individual Techniques
6:00					
11:00					
4:00					
9:00					

FOOD DIARY – Lesson Six

Day of Week _____   Name _____

Time	Minutes Spent Eating	M/S	H	Food Type & Quantity	Individual Techniques
6:00					
11:00					
4:00					
9:00					

FOOD DIARY – Lesson Six

Day of Week _____   Name_____

Time	Minutes Spent Eating	M/S	H	Food Type & Quantity	Individual Techniques
6:00					
11:00					
4:00					
9:00					

FOOD DIARY – Lesson Six

Day of Week _____   Name _____

Time	Minutes Spent Eating	M/S	H	Food Type & Quantity	Individual Techniques
6:00					
11:00					
4:00					
9:00					

FOOD DIARY – Lesson Six

Day of Week _____   Name_____

Time	Minutes Spent Eating	M/S	H	Food Type & Quantity	Individual Techniques
6:00					
11:00					
4:00					
9:00					

FOOD DIARY – Lesson Six

Day of Week _____   Name _____

Time	Minutes Spent Eating	M/S	H	Food Type & Quantity	Individual Techniques
6:00					
11:00					
4:00					
9:00					

FOOD DIARY – Lesson Six

Day of Week _____   Name_____

Time	Minutes Spent Eating	M/S	H	Food Type & Quantity	Individual Techniques
6:00					
11:00					
4:00					
9:00					

DAILY BEHAVIOR CHECKLIST – Lesson Six

Points: Most of the time, or yes = 3
         Sometimes   = 2
         Not at all, or no   = 1

Days of the Week

	1	2	3	4	5	6	7
1. *Daily Checklist* a. Morning Review							
b. Evening scoring							
2. *Food Diary* a. Recording my food							
3. *Cue Elimination* a. Designated eating place							
b. Only eating when eating							
c. Food out of sight							
4. *Eating Delay* a. Utensils down between mouthfuls							
b. Swallowing each forkful before adding the next							
c. Enjoying the meal							
5. *Behavior Chains* a. Break a behavior chain							
b. Substitute an activity for eating							
6. *Pre-planning* a. Pre-plan one or more meals or snacks							
7. *Becoming Your Own Therapist* a. Individual problem solving or working on individual problem							
DAILY TOTALS							

Total Points for the Week _____   Weight _____

BEHAVIORAL PRESCRIPTION SHEET

Name _____

Partner _____

Problem _____
_____
_____
_____

Solutions _____
_____
_____
_____
_____
_____
_____
_____
_____
_____

Plan _____
_____
_____
_____
_____

Feedback _____
_____
_____

Consultation _____

6-14

BEHAVIORAL ANALYSIS AND FEEDBACK FORM

TIME OF EATING

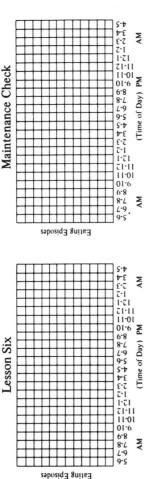

Lesson Six   Maintenance Check

Eating Episodes

(Time of Day)   AM   PM   AM

Indicate the time of day for each eating episode during the week by making a mark in the square above the appropriate time of day. Start with the bottom row of boxes. If you have a second eating episode during the week within that time range, indicate it by filling in the next box in that column. For example, if you had a snack at 10:30 am, you would fill in the first box in the time of day column labeled "10-11 am." If the next day, you had breakfast at 10:15 am, you would blacken in the next box up in that same column. If that same day, you had a snack at 10:50 am, you would indicate this by marking the third box in the same column. When you have entered an entire week's eating pattern in these boxes, you will have a graph which shows the distribution of your eating during the week.

MINUTES SPENT EATING

	Lesson Six		Maintenance Check	
	Meal	Snack	Meal	Snack
0-5 minutes.........				
5-10 minutes......				
10-15 minutes......				
15-20 minutes......				
20-30 minutes......				
over 30 minutes......				

Indicate the duration of *each* of your eating episodes by making a tally mark on the line under the appropriate heading — "meal" or "snack". For example, if breakfast took seven minutes, put a mark under the word "meal" on the line labeled "5-10 minutes." If you had a mid-afternoon snack that lasted 13 minutes, put a mark under "snack" on the line labeled "10-15 minutes." If you had six meals, each 5-10 minutes long, you would have six tallies (卌 l) in the meal column on the line marked 5-10 minutes.

(Adapted from and used by permission of Leonard S. Levitz, Ph.D., and Henry A. Jordan, M.D., University of Pennyslvania School of Medicine, "Analysis of Food Intake and Energy Expenditure," Copyright, 1973.)

BEHAVIORAL ANALYSIS AND FEEDBACK FORM
DEGREE OF HUNGER

	Lesson Six			Maintenance Check	
	Meal	Snack		Meal	Snack
0 – none .... _____	_____	....0 – none .... _____		_____	
1 – some .... _____	_____	....1 – some .... _____		_____	
2 – hungry ... _____	_____	...2 – hungry ... _____		_____	
3 – extreme.. _____	_____	... 3 – extreme .. _____		_____	

Put a tally mark on the appropriate line to indicate the degree of hunger you felt at the beginning of every episode of eating during the week. For example, if you had a snack and were not hungry, put a mark under snack on the line labeled "none." If you felt like you were starving to death when you had dinner, put a mark under "meal" on the line labeled "extreme." (Note: Use the same numbers that appear on your Week One Food Diary.)

BODY POSITION WHILE EATING

	Lesson Six			Maintenance Check	
	Meal	Snack		Meal	Snack
Walking .... _____	_____	Walking .... _____		_____	
Standing ... _____	_____	Standing ... _____		_____	
Sitting ..... _____	_____	Sitting ..... ___ _____		_____	
Lying Down. _____	_____	Lying Down. _____		_____	

Put a tally mark on the appropriate line to indicate your body position during each episode of eating for the week. For example, if you had a snack while walking around the grocery store, put a mark under "snack" on the line labeled "walking". If you ate dinner lying in bed watching television, put a mark under "meal" on the line labeled "lying down."

ACTIVITIES WHILE EATING

	Lesson Six			Maintenance Check	
	Meal	Snack		Meal	Snack
None: only eating .... _____	_____	... _____		_____	
Talking.................. _____	_____	... _____		_____	
Listening to music or radio..... _____	_____	_____		_____	
Reading a book or paper...... _____	_____	... _____		_____	
Watching television.......... _____	_____	... _____		_____	
Cooking-working in kitchen.... _____	_____	... _____		_____	
Working-studying........... _____	_____	... _____		_____	
Other .... _____	_____	... _____		___	___

Put a tally mark on the appropriate line to indicate activities that are associated with your episodes of eating. For example, if you ate lunch while working at your desk, put a mark under "meal" on the line labeled "working." If you had a snack while preparing dinner, put a mark under the "snack" column on the line labeled "cooking."

(Adapted from and used by permission of Leonard S. Levitz, Ph.D., and Henry A. Jordan, M.D., University of Pennsylvania School of Medicine, "Analysis of Food Intake and Energy Expenditure," Copyright, 1973.)

Lesson Seven
CUE ELIMINATION, PART TWO, AND ENERGY USE, PART ONE

7

Lesson Seven
CUE ELIMINATION, PART TWO,
AND ENERGY USE, PART ONE

I.   Weigh-in and Homework.

    A.   Record your weight on your Master Data Sheet.

    B.   The cumulative group average weight loss was _____ .

    C.   Check homework.

        1.   Lesson Six Food Diary.

        2.   Lesson Six Behavior Checklist.

        3.   Pre-planning on the Food Diary.

        4.   Individual problem solving.

    D.   The materials for Lesson Seven include:

        1.   Lesson Seven Outline.

        2.   Lesson Seven Food Diary.

        3.   Lesson Seven Behavior Checklist.

        4.   Daily Activity Sheet.

    E.   For the next four lessons you will need a pedometer. Your leader will loan you one or suggest a place to buy one.

II. Review: Maintenance.

Maintenance of behavior change is fundamental to this weight loss program. The method we have used to build Maintenance into the program is a Behavior Checklist which reminds you of your new behaviors every day. When your new eating skills are solidly established, artificial aids like the checklist can fade out of your daily routine.

Pre-planning

    To change the future, you must plan for it. You will only be able to alter your food intake in a pre-selected direction if you plan ahead. By the time impulse has caught you, it is too late. Pre-planning has a series of steps:

    1.   Designate a time to plan ahead each day.

    2.   Write down your plans and commit yourself.

3.   Correct your pre-planned menu after you eat.

4.   Start by pre-planning one meal or snack, and advance only when you feel you are ready.

5.   If snacks are difficult, pre-prepare them.

6.   Pre-plan party and restaurant eating.

Changing Your Food Buying Behavior

Pre-plan your grocery shopping. Go to the market with a written list of what you are going to buy. Only shop for food after a meal when you are not hungry.

III.   New Technique: Cue Elimination—Part Two (The Starving Armenians).

   A.   Overweight individuals may be more sensitive to environmental cues than their thin counterparts.

   B.   The first cue elimination techniques were aimed at your relationship to your whole environment.   These exercises were:

      1.   Eat only at a designated appropriate eating place.

      2.   Change your habitual eating place at the table.

      3.   When you are eating, only eat—no other activities.

      4.   Work to reduce visual food cues. Remove food from all places in the house other than appropriate storage areas. Store food in opaque containers to keep it out of sight.

      5.   Have alternate foods available to replace empty calorie "junk" or impulse foods.

      6.   Do not leave serving dishes on the table.

   C.   Some of the most difficult cues to eliminate are intimately associated with food.

      1.   Most people are satisfied with less food when the food is served on smaller plates. For this week, try to use smaller plates for your meals when possible.

      2.   We are all conditioned to eat everything on our plates. The reasons for this usually trace back to childhood. "Finish everything on your plate—think of the starving Armenians, Chinese, Europeans, etc.," depending on the era. From now on, leave something behind at every meal.

      3.   If you divide large portions in half, you will be less tempted to finish the second half even though it is available, than if it is all served to you at once. The cognitive or thinking step of asking

yourself, "Do I want seconds?" often will limit you to firsts. This week, divide large portions or meals into halves; after one is eaten, go back for seconds if you are still hungry.

4. Dispose of leftovers. Throw away leftover food. Clear your plates into the disposal, garbage, or pet cat. If something should be saved, pre-plan it into a snack for the next day—but label it for a specific use. Don't let food hang around the house; it will reach out and cue you to eat!

5. Control your food intake. Don't accept food from others unless you ask for it, either at home or at restaurants.

6. Try to minimize contact with food. Put things away and clean up the mess before you sit down to eat the food you prepare.

IV. Energy: Part One (There is No Crisis, Only a Continuing Problem).

A. The second law of thermodynamics cannot be broken by man or beast:

ENERGY IN (food) = ENERGY USED (activity) + STORAGE (fat)

B. So far we have concentrated on the input (food) side of the equation.

C. An increase in energy expenditure or activity plays a vital role in losing weight.

1. It is pleasant not to move around when you are overweight.

2. Regular exercise will accelerate weight loss.

3. Regular exercise can reestablish a weight loss when you have reached a non-losing plateau.

4. An increase in activity often leads to a decrease in appetite. Exercise will cause an increase in appetite only when you are working like a lumberjack.

5. 250 calories additional energy use each day will result in an extra one-half pound weight loss each week, or 26 pounds a year.

D. This week we want to observe your current level of energy expenditure.

1. Record the number of minutes of physical activity and type of activity on the activity sheet in the packet each day. Don't worry about computing calories for now.

2. Write the number of miles recorded by your pedometer on the activity sheet each night. Don't forget to reset it to zero for the next day.

E. To work the pedometer, set the stride by pacing off a measured 100 feet. Divide 100 by the number of steps. This will tell you the length of your average step. For example, if you take 50 steps when you walk 100 feet, your stride is two feet. (100 feet divided by 50 steps equals two feet per step.)

Adjust the stride dial on the pedometer to this number, then firmly clip the pedometer to your belt. The pendulum in the pedometer will click every time you take a step and will automatically register the number of miles you walk. Remember to reset it each evening after you record the total number of miles for the day.

V. Homework.

A. Complete the Lesson Seven Food Diary.

B. Continue pre-planning at least one meal or snack a day.

C. Fill in your Behavior Checklist every day. It includes today's cue elimination exercises:

1. Use smaller plates when possible.

2. Leave food behind on the plate at each meal.

3. Split large meals into seconds.

4. Throw away leftovers immediately after a meal, or label them and pre-plan to use them for a specific meal or snack in the future.

5. Don't accept food from others.

6. Minimize your contacts with food.

D. Write down the number of miles you walk each day and the minutes and type of exercise you engage in during the week on your Daily Activity Sheet.

FOOD DIARY – Lesson Seven

Day of Week_____   Name _____

Time	M/S	Location	Activity While Eating	Food Type and Quantity
6:00				
11:00				
4:00				
9:00				

FOOD DIARY – Lesson Seven

Day of Week_____   Name _____

Time	M/S	Location	Activity While Eating	Food Type and Quantity
6:00				
11:00				
4:00				
9:00				

FOOD DIARY – Lesson Seven

Day of Week_____   Name_____

Time	M/S	Location	Activity While Eating	Food Type and Quantity
6:00				
11:00				
4:00				
9:00				

FOOD DIARY – Lesson Seven

Day of Week_____   Name_____

Time	M/S	Location	Activity While Eating	Food Type and Quantity
6:00				
11:00				
4:00				
9:00				

FOOD DIARY – Lesson Seven

Day of Week_____   Name_____

Time	M/S	Location	Activity While Eating	Food Type and Quantity
6:00				
11:00				
4:00				
9:00				

FOOD DIARY – Lesson Seven

Day of Week_____   Name_____

Time	M/S	Location	Activity While Eating	Food Type and Quantity
6:00				
11:00				
4:00				
9:00				

FOOD DIARY — Lesson Seven

Day of Week_____   Name_____

Time	M/S	Location	Activity While Eating	Food Type and Quantity
6:00				
11:00				
4:00				
9:00				

DAILY BEHAVIOR CHECKLIST — Lesson Seven

Points: Most of the time, or yes = 3
Sometimes = 2
Not at all, or no = 1

				Days			
	1	2	3	4	5	6	7
1. *Daily Checklist* a. Morning Review							
b. Evening Scoring							
2. *Food Diary* a. Recording my food							
3. *Cue Elimination – I* a. Designated eating place							
b. Only eating when eating							
4. *Eating Delay* a. Swallow each forkful before adding the next							
5. *Behavior Chains* a. Substitute an activity for eating							
6. *Pre-planning* a. Pre-plan one or more meals or snacks							
b. Shop on a full stomach							
7. *Cue Elimination – II* a. Use smaller plates when possible							
b. Leave food behind on the plate							
c. Split large meals into seconds							
d. Throw away or commit leftovers							
e. Don't accept food from others							
f. Minimize your contact with food.							
Daily Totals							

Total Points for the Week _____   Weight _____

DAILY ACTIVITY SHEET

(Fill in miles per day walked and minutes of exercise or extra activities)

	Monday		Tuesday		Wednesday		Thursday		Friday		Saturday		Sunday	
	Miles	Calories	Miles	Calories	Miles	Calories	Miles	Calories	Miles	Calories	Miles	Calories	Miles	Calories
Miles Walked														
	Mins.	Calories	Mins.	Calories	Mins.	Calories	Mins.	Calories	Mins.	Calories	Mins.	Calories	Mins.	Calories
Activity or Exercise														

Lesson Eight
ENERGY USE, PART TWO

8

Lesson Eight
ENERGY USE, PART TWO

I.   Weigh-in and Homework.

    A.   Record your weight on your Master Data Sheet.

    B.   The cumulative group average weight loss was _____.

    C.   Homework.

        1.   Lesson Seven Food Diary.

        2.   Pre-planning written on Food Diary.

        3.   Lesson Seven Behavior Checklist.

        4.   Miles per day recorded on the Daily Activity Sheet.

        5.   Minutes of exercise on the Daily Activity Sheet.

    D.   The materials for Lesson Eight include:

        1.   Lesson Eight Outline.

        2.   Lesson Eight Food Diary.

        3.   Lesson Eight Behavior Checklist.

        4.   Daily Activity Sheet.

        5.   Table of "Calories Burned Up."

        6.   Daily Energy-Out (activity) Graph.

II.   Review: Cue Elimination—Part Two.

Six techniques were introduced last lesson to help you start to eliminate cues that are inherent in eating situations. In many ways these cues are more difficult to eliminate than remote environmental cues. You can walk away from the television to eat a lamb chop, but you cannot walk away from the lamb chop and still eat it. The techniques suggested were:

    1.   Use smaller plates. This will give a realistic illusion of more food when compared with the same amount on a large plate.

    2.   Consciously leave food behind on the plate and start to break up that conditioned need to clean up your plate. Stop feeding that starving Armenian inside you.

    3.   Divide large portions into two halves to put a thinking break in the middle of a meal. You have to think about food quantity to go back for seconds.

4.   Throw away or plan a use for leftovers and scraps. If you keep them, label them and pre-plan them for a specific use. This will eliminate a lot of the food that is commonly used for snacks. Leftovers are very potent cues for eating.

5.   Don't accept food from others—ask for what you want at home and in restaurants.

6.   Minimize your contact with food. When you are preparing food, cleanup the mess before you sit down to eat. This will make it harder to go back for seconds.

III.   Energy Use: Part Two—(The Continuing Crisis).

A.   The second law of thermodynamics can be paraphrased:

ENERGY IN (food) = ENERGY USED (activity) + STORAGE (fat);

or,

STORAGE (fat) = ENERGY IN (food) − ENERGY USED (activity)

We are governed by the same laws that rule the universe—there are no exceptions for man or beast.

B.   The first seven lessons have concentrated on the ENERGY IN side of the equation by decreasing the amount of unnecessary and impulse food you eat.

C.   Increasing activity or using more energy has many advantages:
1.   Your muscle tone will improve with increased activity, and your weight loss will be primarily from fat stores.

2.   Exercise might break up some of the emotional cues such as boredom or the blues that lead to excessive eating.

3.   Hard exercise will often decrease your appetite, especially for an immediately succeeding meal.

4.   As you lose weight, your body will regain a thin athletic shape.

5.   Your body tone will improve, and your cardiovascular system will be more proficient.

6.   You will enjoy life more.

D.   You use energy in four distinct ways during a day's activity:

1.   The Basal Metabolic Rate is the basic energy requirement to maintain your body in a warm, alive state. It is affected by a great many factors and is not fixed throughout your life.

2. About seven percent of your intake is used to digest your food.

3. All physical activity uses up energy. Even standing uses more than sitting.

4. Energy is stored when you consume more than you burn. This storage is in high energy deposits of fat.

E. How many calories do you need each day?

1. The caloric requirements for the body weight maintenance for the average weight American adult is:

(Age)	22-35	35-55	55-75
Men	2800	2600	2400
Women	2000	1850	1700

2. Outside of the normal weight range, you can very roughly estimate the number of calories needed to maintain your weight by multiplying your body weight by 15.

3. One pound of body fat loss is equal to 3500 calories consumed, burned up, or both.

F. COMMIT HERESY TODAY—WASTE ENERGY; expend more energy every chance you get.

1. You can increase your energy use by including more exercise in your daily life, or by increasing your everyday activities and becoming more wasteful. Sit instead of lying down, stand instead of sit, walk instead of drive, take stairs instead of elevators. Or add some new activities, like a sport or a regular walk in the neighborhood.

2. The goal of this exercise is to burn 250 extra calories every day. This is a distant goal and should be approached in steps appropriate for you.

IV. Assignment.

A. Increase normal activities.

1. Answer the phone farthest away (but still close enough to get the message).

2. Use the farthest bathroom at home and work.

3. Park the car at the end of the parking lot or a block away from where you are going. (Remember to leave earlier for your appointment.)

4. Stand as much as possible.

5. Use stairs instead of elevators.

6. Walk rather than drive when possible.

7. Meet the bus farther away.

8. Be creative.

B. Keep wearing your pedometer. Graph the number of miles you walk each day. Use the techniques introduced today and try to increase your mileage by 50 percent this week.

C. Increase your exercise.

1. Choose some activity you like to do.

2. Start out slowly and avoid strains.

3. If possible, exercise with someone.

4. Be active!

D. Estimate the number of extra calories you spend each day, graph it, and try to increase it by 50 or 100 calories during the next week.

V. Recipes (optional).

VI. Homework.

A. Lesson Eight Food Diary.

B. Lesson Eight Behavior Checklist.

C. Daily Activity Sheet.

D. Daily Energy-Out (activity) Graph.

VII. For the next lesson, you will need a pocket calorie counter. These are available at most bookstores, markets, and drug stores for a low cost. Your group leader can suggest places to buy them.

FOOD DIARY – Lesson Eight

Day of Week _____   Name_____

Time	M/S	H	Location of Eating	Food Type and Quantity
6:00				
11:00				
4:00				
9:00				

FOOD DIARY – Lesson Eight

Day of Week _____   Name _____

Time	M/S	H	Location of Eating	Food Type and Quantity
6:00				
11:00				
4:00				
9:00				

FOOD DIARY – Lesson Eight

Day of Week _____   Name_____

Time	M/S	H	Location of Eating	Food Type and Quantity
6:00				
11:00				
4:00				
9:00				

FOOD DIARY – Lesson Eight

Day of Week _____   Name _____

Time	M/S	H	Location of Eating	Food Type and Quantity
6:00				
11:00				
4:00				
9:00				

FOOD DIARY – Lesson Eight

Day of Week _____   Name _____

Time	M/S	H	Location of Eating	Food Type and Quantity
6:00				
11:00				
4:00				
9:00				

FOOD DIARY – Lesson Eight

Day of Week _____   Name_____

Time	M/S	H	Location of Eating	Food Type and Quantity
6:00				
11:00				
4:00				
9:00				

FOOD DIARY – Lesson Eight

Day of Week _____   Name _____

Time	M/S	H	Location of Eating	Food Type and Quantity
6:00				
11:00				
4:00				
9:00				

DAILY BEHAVIOR CHECKLIST — Lesson 8

Points: Most of the time, or yes = 3
         Sometimes   = 2
         Not at all, or no   = 1

Days of the Week

	1	2	3	4	5	6	7
1. *Daily Checklist*							
a. Morning review							
b. Evening scoring							
2. *Food Diary*							
a. Recording my food							
3. *Cue Elimination — I*							
a. Designated eating place							
b. Food stored in opaque container							
4. *Pre-planning*							
a. Pre-plan one or more meals or snacks							
b. Shop from a prepared list							
5. *Cue Elimination — II*							
a. Leave food behind on the plate							
b. Split large meals into seconds							
c. Throw away or label leftovers							
d. Don't accept food from others							
6. *Energy Use*							
a. Record miles walked per day							
b. Increase miles walked per day							
c. Increase other activities							
DAILY TOTALS							

Total Points for the Week _____   Weight _____

DAILY ACTIVITY SHEET

(Fill in miles per day walked and minutes of exercise or extra activities)

	Monday		Tuesday		Wednesday		Thursday		Friday		Saturday		Sunday	
	Miles	Calories	Miles	Calories	Miles	Calories	Miles	Calories	Miles	Calories	Miles	Calories	Miles	Calories
Miles Walked														
	Mins.	Calories	Mins.	Calories	Mins.	Calories	Mins.	Calories	Mins.	Calories	Mins.	Calories	Mins.	Calories
Activity or Exercise														

CALORIES BURNED UP DURING TEN MINUTES OF CONTINUOUS ACTIVITY

	Body Wt.#	150#	175#	200#	225#	250#	275#	300#
PERSONAL ACTIVITIES								
Sleeping		12	14	16	18	20	22	24
Sitting (TV or reading)		12	14	16	18	20	22	24
Sitting (Conversing)		18	21	24	28	30	34	37
Washing/Dressing		32	38	42	47	53	58	63
Standing quietly		14	17	19	21	24	26	28
SEDENTARY OCCUPATION								
Sitting/Writing		18	21	24	28	30	34	37
Light Office Work		30	35	39	45	50	55	60
Standing (Light activity)		24	28	32	37	40	45	50
HOUSEWORK								
General Housework		41	48	53	60	68	74	81
Washing Windows		42	49	54	61	69	76	83
Making Beds		39	46	52	58	65	75	85
Mopping Floors		46	54	60	68	75	83	91
Light Gardening		36	42	47	53	59	66	73
Weeding Garden		59	69	78	88	98	109	120
Mowing Grass (power)		41	48	53	60	67	74	81
Mowing Grass (manual)		45	53	58	66	74	81	88
Shoveling Snow		78	92	100	117	130	144	160
LIGHT WORK								
Factory Assembly		24	28	32	37	40	45	50
Truck-Auto Repair		42	49	54	61	69	76	83
Carpentry/Farm Work		38	45	51	58	64	71	78
Brick Laying		34	40	45	51	57	62	67
HEAVY WORK								
Chopping Wood		73	86	96	109	121	134	156
Pick & Shovel Work		67	79	88	100	110	120	130

CALORIES BURNED UP DURING TEN MINUTES OF CONTINUOUS ACTIVITY (Continued)

	Body Wt.#	150#	175#	200#	225#	250#	275#	300#
LOCOMOTION								
Walking - 2 mph		35	40	46	53	58	64	69
One mile - @ 2 mph		105	120	140	157	175	193	210
Walking - 4-1/2 mph		67	78	87	98	110	120	131
One mile - @ 4-1/2 mph		89	103	115	130	147	160	173
Walking Upstairs		175	201	229	259	288	318	350
Walking Downstairs		67	78	88	100	111	122	134
Jogging - 5-1/2 mph		108	127	142	160	178	197	215
Running - 7 mph		141	164	187	208	232	256	280
Running - 12 mph (sprint)		197	230	258	295	326	360	395
Running in place (140 count)		242	284	325	363	405	447	490
Bicycle - 5-1/2 mph		50	58	67	75	83	92	101
Bicycle - 13 mph		107	125	142	160	178	197	216
RECREATION								
Badminton or Vollyball		52	67	75	85	94	104	115
Baseball (except pitcher)		47	54	62	70	78	86	94
Basketball		70	82	93	105	117	128	140
Bowling (nonstop)		67	82	90	100	111	122	133
Canadian Airforce								
Exercise -0.5 Bx 1A		83	97	108	123	137	152	168
2A		104	122	137	155	173	190	207
3A,4A		147	170	192	217	244	267	290
5A,6A		167	192	217	240	270	300	330
Dancing - moderate		42	49	55	62	69	77	86
Dancing - vigorous		57	67	75	86	94	104	115
Square Dancing		68	80	90	103	113	124	135
Football		83	97	110	123	137	152	167
Golf - foursome		40	47	55	62	68	75	83
Horseback Riding (trot)		67	78	90	102	112	123	134
Ping Pong		38	43	52	58	64	71	78
Skiing - (alpine)		96	113	128	145	160	177	195
Skiing - (cross country)		117	137	158	174	194	214	235
Skiing - (water)		73	92	104	117	130	142	165
Swimming - (backstroke)								
20 yd/min		38	43	52	58	64	71	79
Swimming - (breaststroke)								
20 yd/min		48	55	63	72	80	88	96
Swimming-crawl 20 yd/min		48	55	63	72	80	88	96
Tennis		67	80	92	103	115	125	135
Wrestling, Judo or Karate		129	150	175	192	213	235	257

DAILY ENERGY-OUT (ACTIVITY) GRAPH

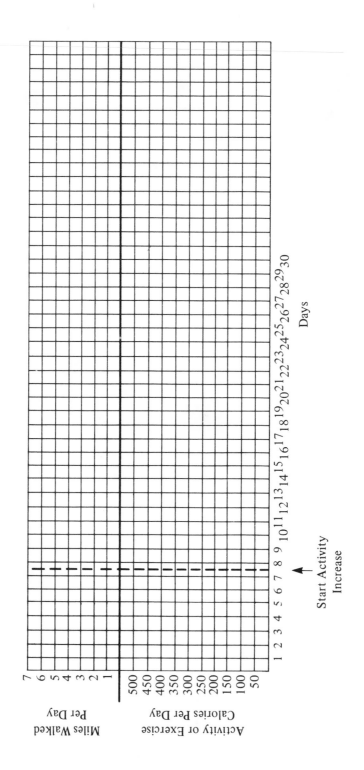

Lesson Nine
SNACKS, CUES, AND HOLIDAYS

Lesson Nine
SNACKS, CUES AND
HOLIDAYS

I.   Weigh-in and Homework.

    A.   Record your weight on the Master Data Sheet.

    B.   The cumulative group average weight loss was_____ .

    C.   Homework.

        1.   Lesson Eight Food Diary.

        2.   Pre-planning written on the Food Diary.

        3.   Lesson Eight Behavior Checklist.

        4.   Miles per day recorded on your Daily Activity Sheet.

        5.   Miles per day graphed.

        6.   Minutes per day of activities recorded.

    D.   The materials for Lesson Nine include:

        1.   Lesson Nine Outline.

        2.   Daily Activity Sheet.

        3.   Snack Worksheet.

        4.   Maintenance Behavior Checklist.

        5.   Optional Food Diary.

    E.   Next lesson is family night. If possible bring a spouse, friend, child, or anyone who is interested in your weight control and eating behavior change program. We will go over some of the topics covered in the course and point out some of the ways others can help you with Maintenance after the course has ended.

II.   Review: Pre-planning.

Habitually pre-planning meals and restricting your food intake to what you have planned is one of the strongest ways of counteracting impulse eating.

    Change your food buying habits by pre-planning your shopping, and go to the market on a full stomach.

Cue Elimination

    A.   The first set of cue elimination exercises was designed to lessen the effect of environmental cues on eating behaviors. Now, after several months of practice, these cue elimination exercises should be habitual. You should be able to feel the difference, to be aware of the reduced strength of old food cues like television.

    B.   The second set of cue elimination exercises must be practiced every day until they become habit:

        1.   Leave food behind at the end of each meal or snack.

        2.   Throw away or pre-plan leftovers—get them out of your life.

        3.   Divide large portions into two halves.

        4.   Use smaller plates and shallower bowls.

        5.   Don't accept food from others.

        6.   Try to minimize your contact with food. Clean up before you eat your meal.

Energy—Its Use and Abuse

    A.   If you use more energy than you consume, you will lose weight.

    B.   Increasing everyday activity is the easiest way to use up more energy. One extra mile walked every day will result in 12 pounds of weight loss in a year without any change in your food intake.

    C.   The goal last week was a 50 percent increase in daily mileage and 50-100 extra activity calories burned up every day.

    D.   The goal by next week is 250 extra calories used up per day (one-half extra pound lost per week) through increased daily activity.

III.   New Topic: Snacks and Holiday Control.

    A.   Snacks are usually the result of impulse, a response to a non-physiologic, non-hunger cue. These cues are situation specific and time limited.

    B.   Impulse eating is especially a problem under two conditions:

        1.   Holidays, where the environment is saturated with eating cues.

        2.   During ordinary meals. This includes anything eaten after you cannot answer the question, "Am I hungry" with a "yes"—it might be an extra chop, a piece of bread, or a larger dessert.

C.   If you can control the impulse to eat when you are not hungry, you will dramatically decrease your daily caloric intake.

D.   We have introduced many techniques that can be used to control snacking. These will be your first line of defense during holidays, vacations, and other times when there is an increased probability of snacking or impulsive eating.

    1.   Build time delays into snacks—put ten minutes between your urge and your snack.

    2.   Slow down, put your food down and take time to enjoy each bite.

    3.   Eat at your designated appropriate eating place.

    4.   Substitute alternate behaviors for eating.

    5.   Pre-plan your food and drink intake.

    6.   Do all shopping on a full stomach from a list. Don't buy snack foods.

    7.   Leave some part of each food type behind. Throw it away. Control your environment, don't let it control you.

E.   Physiology and psychology experiments have demonstrated that people cannot sense calories.

    1.   People feel full when they consume a large volume of food.

    2.   People feel full when they believe they have eaten high-calorie food.

    3.   Your sensitivity to volume can be used to advantage. If you feed your hunger pangs with volume instead of calories, or something that carries with it the illusion of calories, such as diet candy, you will find hunger pangs will be satisfied. Cued or psychological hunger is short-lived. If it is not rewarded with food, it will go away.

    4.   Start your meals and snacks with volume—water, diet drinks, salad, celery, etc., and stop eating when you are no longer hungry.

    5.   Don't forget your old cue elimination exercises.

F.   Food Substitutions .

    1.   The calorie content of food is not intuitively obvious—to find out the calorie worth of many foods, you must consult a calorie book.

    2.   In many situations you have a choice of foods, hors d'oeuvres, meals or snacks. If you know how much they are worth, you

can make an informed decision about which one to eat. For example, if you go to a graduation dinner and have a choice between 3-1/2 ounces of duck and 3-1/2 ounces of lobster for a main course, it will help you make the decision if you know the duck contains 350 calories and the lobster only 95.

3. Among the materials for today you will find a Snack Worksheet. Fill in snacks from your Food Diary for last week, choose a substitute snack from your calorie counter, and calculate your potential savings.

IV. New Forms: The Cues.

A. The Food Diary is optional this week.

B. The Maintenance Behavior Checklist will be your Maintenance tool. It should be used in two ways:

1. Use it as a cueing device. Read it before each meal to remind you of the behaviors you have learned.

2. Use it as a recording and self-evaluation or feedback device. Each evening, check your behaviors for the day. Keep track of how well you are maintaining the behaviors on the list. If your performance begins to fall off, go back to the lesson that taught that behavior and relearn it.

V. Homework.

A. Continue to fill in the Daily Activity Sheet for the coming week. Try to reach 250 calories of energy used up above your baseline every day for the coming week. This will be the combined total energy spent in walking and other forms of exercising.

B. Fill in your Daily Energy-Out Graph with information from your Daily Activity Sheet.

C. Fill in the Maintenance Behavior Checklist every day.

D. The Food Diary is optional.

E. Bring a family member or friend next week.

SNACK HINTS

1. Make snacks hard to get. They should require preparation, like popcorn, or be hard to eat, like frozen banannas.

2. Try to avoid extremes of intake — neither starvation nor over-eating — they both lead to feast/famine cycles, and extra eating between meals. Never skip a meal if you're hungry — eat with control.

3. High protein foods will decrease food cravings — they last longer.

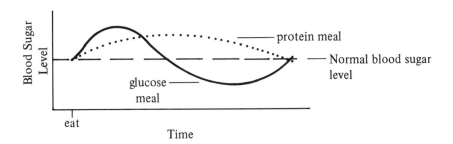

3. A small glass of unsweetened orange juice will help you overcome that famished feeling — combine it with a high protein snack if necessary.

4. Caffeine lowers blood sugar and stimulates hunger.

5. Alcohol is caloric, stimulates hunger and leads to higher levels of blood triglycerides.

6. Use unsaturated fats when possible (especially men).

7. Read labels. Some artificial creamers use coconut (saturated fat) oils instead of corn oil and may contain more calories. Diet colas vary from 2 to 72 calories per can. Water-packed foods have many fewer calories than syrup-packed. The order in which contents are listed on labels indicate how much of each is present inside the container. For example — the Cheerios label says it contains oat flour, wheat starch, *sugar*, salt, sodium phosphate. Sugar is the third most prevalent constituent of Cheerios.

8. Carry a low-calorie sweetner with you.

9. If quantity is your weakness, add bulk; for example, raw vegetables, long grain rice, a diet soda before dinner, or starting dinner with boullion for a soup course.

10. Try to always have an alternate response to snack eating — and keep in mind, a little hunger is the feeling of losing weight.

SNACK WORKSHEET

For This Food	Substitute	Savings

FOOD DIARY – Lesson Nine
  (OPTIONAL)

Day of Week _____   Name _____

Time	M/S	H	Food Type and Quantity
6:00			
11:00			
4:00			
9:00			

FOOD DIARY – Lesson Nine
(OPTIONAL)

Day of Week _____ __   Name _____

Time	M/S	H	Food Type and Quantity
6:00			
11:00			
4:00			
9:00			

FOOD DIARY – Lesson Nine
     (OPTIONAL)

Day of Week _____   Name _____

Time	M/S	H	Food Type and Quantity
6:00			
11:00			
4:00			
9:00			

FOOD DIARY – Lesson Nine
(OPTIONAL)

Day of Week _____   Name _____

Time	M/S	H	Food Type and Quantity
6:00			
11:00			
4:00			
9:00			

FOOD DIARY – Lesson Nine
   (OPTIONAL)

Day of Week ————————   Name ————————————

Time	M/S	H	Food Type and Quantity
6:00			
11:00			
4:00			
9:00			

FOOD DIARY – Lesson Nine
(OPTIONAL)

Day of Week _____   Name _____

Time	M/S	H	Food Type and Quantity
6:00			
11:00			
4:00			
9:00			

FOOD DIARY – Lesson Nine
(OPTIONAL)

Day of Week _____   Name _____

Time	M/S	H	Food Type and Quantity
6:00			
11:00			
4:00			
9:00			

DAILY ACTIVITY SHEET

(Fill in miles per day walked and minutes of exercise or extra activities)

	Monday		Tuesday		Wednesday		Thursday		Friday		Saturday		Sunday	
	Miles	Calories	Miles	Calories	Miles	Calories	Miles	Calories	Miles	Calories	Miles	Calories	Miles	Calories
Miles Walked														
	Mins.	Calories	Mins.	Calories	Mins.	Calories	Mins.	Calories	Mins.	Calories	Mins.	Calories	Mins.	Calories
Activity or Exercise														

MAINTENANCE BEHAVIOR CHECKLIST – WEEK ____

√ : Good Job

	Wt.		Days					
		1	2	3	4	5	6	7
Designated eating place								
No other activity while eating								
Utensils down between mouthfuls								
Smaller plates and shallow bowls								
Leave food behind								
Dispose of (or pre-plan) leftovers								
Store food out of sight								
Minimize contact with food								
Substitute activities for eating								
Increase exercise								
Increase walking								
Pre-plan meals & snacks								
Only eat what you need!								
Take time and enjoy your meals								
No. of √'s ____								

9-16

Lesson Ten
ENVIRONMENTAL SUPPORT—FAMILY AND FRIENDS

10

Lesson Ten
ENVIRONMENTAL SUPPORT–
FAMILY AND FRIENDS

I. Weigh-in.

    A. Weigh the group members, record their weights, and have them graph their weight change.

    B. The cumulative group average weight loss was _____ .

    C. The materials for Lesson Ten include:

        1. Lesson Ten Outline.

        2. Maintenance Behavior Checklist.

        3. Optional Food Diary.

        4. Recipes and food hints from the group (optional).

    D. Today you will receive your contingent refund. The money you have earned by doing your homework.

    E. Return your pedometer and calorie counter if they were on loan from the group leader.

II. Environmental Support.

We invited your family and friends today for several reasons. We want to provide information and tell them what this mysterious program of weight control has been about. In the next hour we will review the program, both in theory and practice, and discuss the progress made by the group. Then we will discuss the role of your social environment, the important people around you, and how these people can help you control your weight and maintain your new eating behavior patterns.

    An individual's social environment provides his or her major source of reward or reinforcement and feedback about progress and success. If people close to you do not know what is going on, what you are trying to change, it is difficult for them to react appropriately to any changes you make. You need their support, cooperation, and encouragement to maintain your behavior changes and weight loss.

III. Review: Activity.

An equation can be written to describe the process of weight gain and loss.

$$\text{ENERGY IN (FOOD)} = \text{ENERGY USED (ACTIVITY)} + \text{STORAGE (FAT)}$$

or,

$$\text{FAT} = \text{FOOD} - \text{ACTIVITY}$$

Last week we proposed you increase your total activity expenditure by 250 calories per day over your original activity level. This will use 1750 extra calories a week, the equivalent of one-half pound. This can be accomplished by being more energetic, or wasteful of energy, in everyday activities, and by including additional activities in your regular routine.

Snacks, Cues and Holidays

A. Many of the techniques we have introduced in this course apply to impulse eating. Last week we reviewed the techniques that are applicable to snacking. The impulse to eat can also be reduced by the use of bulk in your diet, because you are apt to feel satisfied when you feel your stomach is full.

B. Much holiday eating and snacking is in a social context where you have a choice between foods. If you know the caloric content of snack or impulse items, you can choose a lower-calorie food. The caloric content of foods is not intuitively obvious, so we provided a calorie worksheet, and suggested you buy an inexpensive calorie counter.

General Review

1. The theory behind the course and the Food Diary.

2. The concept and practice of cue elimination.

3. Putting delays in your eating and enjoying what you eat.

4. Solving problems and becoming your own therapist.

5. Pre-planning: a way to avoid impulse eating.

IV. New Topic: The Social Environment—Spouse, Family, and Friends.

A. Interactions with others concerning weight loss tend to follow patterns; some of the negative feelings perceived by people losing weight are:

1. "No one is interested in what I am doing."

2. "No one supports my change."

3. "People discourage me."

4. "My efforts are ignored."

5. "My loss is praised, but Maintenance is ignored."

6. "I am being sabotaged."

B. Many reasons can be suggested to explain these interactions. The most probable one is that this is just a way that individuals around you have learned to interact with you when you are losing weight. Any social environment includes many behaviors and habitual interactions that have persisted for a long time, without either person being fully aware of what is occurring between them. The more you can involve others in your weight loss program, the fewer of these negative interactions you will have. Many can be avoided by being prepared for them.

C. To break out of these stereotyped interactions, most of the responsibility must be undertaken by the person losing weight:

1. Ask for what you want—praise, feedback, cooperation, and reward.

2. Ask for help with the techniques.

3. Request that affection and sharing not be associated with food.

4. Ask people not to offer you food; assure them you will ask for what you want to eat.

5. Minimize "food talk" when you are with friends; it is a social cue to eat.

6. Entertain without high-calorie foods.

7. Ask people not to snack around you; they will cue you to eat or be hungry.

8. Try to develop exercise programs with others.

V. Maintenance.

You should fill out your Maintenance Behavior Checklist for the next six weeks. Read it before each meal to remind yourself of the behaviors, and fill it out each evening to evaluate your Maintenance. One copy of an optional Food Diary is included for use in case you find yourself losing your new behaviors or gaining weight.

Next week, or next year, go back to the Food Diaries. Find out what the problems are, and review the appropriate part of the program. In many cases reintroducing the Food Diary will be sufficient to reestablish all of your new eating skills. If you want to analyze your eating behaviors either now or in the future, keep a detailed (Lesson 4) Food Diary for one week. When it is completed, turn back to Lesson Six and fill in the remaining half of the Behavioral Analysis Form. This will give you a good picture of how well your behaviors are being maintained and what areas need improvement.

We will have weekly Maintenance sessions for the next five weeks. They are optional. If you come, bring your Maintenance Behavior checklist so we can help solve any problems that come up.

FOOD DIARY – Lesson Ten
(OPTIONAL)

Day of Week _____   Name _____

Time	M/S	H	Food Type and Quantity
6:00			
11:00			
4:00			
9:00			

MAINTENANCE BEHAVIOR CHECKLIST – WEEK ____

√ : Good Job

	Wt.	Days						
		1	2	3	4	5	6	7
Designated eating place								
No other activity while eating								
Utensils down between mouthfuls								
Smaller plates and shallow bowls								
Leave food behind								
Dispose of (or pre-plan) leftovers								
Store food out of sight								
Minimize contact with food								
Substitute activities for eating								
Increase exercise								
Increase walking								
Pre-plan meals & snacks								
Only eat what you need!								
Take time and enjoy your meals								
No. of √'s ____								